REVIEW OF NEURORADIOLOGY

VAL M. RUNGE, M.D.

Rosenbaum Professor of Radiology
University of Kentucky
College of Medicine
Chandler Medical Center
Lexington, Kentucky

W.B. SAUNDERS COMPANY
A Division of Harcourt Brace & Company
Philadelphia London Toronto Montreal Sydney Tokyo

W.B. SAUNDERS COMPANY
A Division of Harcourt Brace & Company

The Curtis Center
Independence Square West
Philadelphia, Pennsylvania 19106

Library of Congress Cataloging-in-Publication Data

Runge, Val M.
    Review of neuroradiology / Val M. Runge. — 1st ed.

      p.   cm.

    ISBN 0-7216-5134-8

    1. Nervous system—Radiography.   I. Title.
    [DNLM: 1. Neuroradiography.   2. Diagnostic Imaging.   3. Diagnostic
Imaging.   4. Central Nervous System—physiopathology.   5. Central
Nervous System Diseases—diagnosis.   WL 141 R942r 1995]
    RC349.R3R86   1996
    616.8'04757—dc20

DNLM/DLC   95-19483

REVIEW OF NEURORADIOLOGY   ISBN 0-7216-5134-8

Printed in the United States of America.

Last digit is the print number: 9 8 7 6 5 4 3 2 1

To Valerie, Sadie, and B.J.,
With All My Love

P R E F A C E

This text is designed to be used in preparation for either the Neuroradiology subsection of the board exam or the Neuroradiology subspecialty exam. It also serves as an excellent concise review of Neuroradiology, with an emphasis on MR, for those wishing an update. The use of MR is covered in greater depth than that of CT, angiography, and myelography, due to the dominance of this modality in current clinical practice and the need for continuing medical education. The subject matter is divided along classic lines into three major divisions: skull and contents (brain), head and neck, and spine. To assist in use as a reference source, all sections are coded according to the *Index for Radiological Diagnoses,* 4th edition, as published by the American College of Radiology (ACR). This provides both an excellent organizational framework as well as a quick method for reference. For those not familiar with the ACR code, these numbers can be ignored. To avoid being wordy, information is conveyed in short phrases, as opposed to sentences. The text is equally well suited to be read from cover to cover or to be used as a reference source for specific topics.

Val M. Runge, M.D.

CONTENTS

SKULL AND CONTENTS (BRAIN)

Magnetic Resonance Technique ....

1.121411

Spin-echo technique

- basics

    90° radiofrequency (RF) pulse followed by 180° RF pulse

    generates signal "echo" at time TE

    TE = time interval between 90° pulse and spin-echo signal

    magnetic resonance (MR) signal decreases with increasing TE

    differences between tissues based on T_2 values—maximized at long TE

    pulsing repeated at intervals of TR

    TR = time interval between successive 90°–180° RF pulse pairs

    differences between tissues based on T_1 values—maximized at short TR

- T_1-weighted

    short TR, TE (<500, <25, respectively)

    high intrinsic tissue contrast

    fat is high signal intensity (SI) (bright or white), cerebrospinal fluid (CSF) is low SI (dark or black), gray matter is slightly hypointense to white matter

    = longitudinal (spin-lattice) relaxation time

        refers to time required for tissue magnetization to return to thermal equilibrium

        short T_1—faster magnetization recovery

        increases with magnetic field strength

- T_2-weighted

    long TR, TE (>2000, >45, respectively)

    high intrinsic tissue contrast

    fat is low SI (dark), CSF is high SI (bright), gray matter is slightly hyperintense to white matter

    = transverse (spin-spin) relaxation time

        refers to time required for magnetization in transverse plane to dephase and lose coherence

        short T_2—faster dephasing

        relatively independent of magnetic field strength

- Proton (spin) density

    long TR, short TE (>2000, <25, respectively)

    poor intrinsic tissue contrast, high signal-to-noise ratio (SNR)

    = number of hydrogen nuclei/unit volume tissue

Fast spin-echo technique

- multiple spin echoes generated following each 90° RF pulse (by repeating the 180° pulse), with each echo used to acquire additional phase-encoding steps

- typically employed for T_2-weighting
- comparison with spin echo
  - fat is higher SI
  - less susceptibility effect
  - increased RF deposition
  - substantially reduced scan times
    - can be employed to improve image quality or to improve spatial resolution

---

1.121412

Spoiled gradient-echo (GRE) technique (= FLASH = SP GRASS)

- nomenclature
  - FLASH = fast low = angle shot
  - SP-GRASS = spoiled gradient-recalled acquisition in the steady state
- longitudinal magnetization is allowed to approach steady state
- transverse magnetization is "spoiled" away (before subsequent RF pulsing), and does not contribute to observed signal
- comparison to spin-echo technique
  - similar in regard to signal generation and contrast
  - no 180° RF pulse employed—echo created by use of gradients
  - additional dependency of contrast on RF flip angle
  - T_2^* dependency—due to absence of 180° RF pulse (also increased sensitivity to magnetic field inhomogeneities, metal)
- contrast dependency
  - at RF flip angle of 90°, same as spin echo (except T_2^* effects)
  - at reduced flip angle (<90°)
    - similar contrast to spin echo, but with shorter TR
    - SNR advantage vs. spin echo at very short TR
  - at very small flip angles—T_2^*-weighting achieved
- utility—provides good T_1 contrast
  - rapid 2-D imaging
  - high resolution 3-D imaging in reasonable scan time

Rephased gradient-echo (GRE) technique (= FISP = FAST = GRASS)

- nomenclature
  - FISP = fast imaging with steady precession
  - FAST = Fourier-acquired steady state
  - GRASS = gradient-recalled acquisition in steady state
- a steady-state free precession (SSFP) technique, with observation of SSFP free induction decay (FID) signal—thus a T_2 depen-dency
- longitudinal and transverse magnetization approach steady state

- comparison to spin-echo technique

    no 180° RF pulse employed—echo created by use of gradients

    additional dependency of contrast on RF flip angle

    T_2^* dependency—due to absence of 180° RF pulse (also increased sensitivity to magnetic field inhomogeneities, metal)

- contrast dependency

    at long TR (300 msec), similar contrast to spoiled GRE regardless of flip angle

    at short TR (30 msec)

        small flip angle—T_2/T_1-(mixed) weighting with loss of gray-white matter differentiation (vs. T_1-weighting of spoiled GRE)

        large flip angle—high water (CSF) SI ("water weighting")

- utility

    rapid 2-D imaging

T_2-enhanced gradient echo (GRE) technique (= CE-FAST = PSIF)

- nomenclature

    CE-FAST = contrast-enhanced Fourier-acquired steady state

    PSIF = time-reversed FISP

- SSFP technique, with observation of SSFP echo signal (FID is not acquired)
- transverse magnetization is maintained
- comparison to spin-echo technique

    no 180° RF pulse employed—echo created by gradients

    T_2^* dependency—due to absence of 180° RF pulse (also increased sensitivity to magnetic field inhomogeneities, metal)

    low SNR

    sensitive to motion and flow artifacts

- contrast dependency

    very short TR, large flip angle—T_2

- utility

    perfusion (first pass) studies

    breathhold 2-D imaging

    3-D imaging

Three-dimensional (3-D) imaging

- basics

    spatial encoding by using the readout gradient in one dimension, and phase-encoding in other *two* dimensions

    comparison with 2-D

        longer imaging time (due to use of second phase-encoding gradient)—reasonable scan times achieved with GRE imaging and short TRs

        true contiguous sections—no slice-to-slice interference, better thin section capabilities

- utility

  allows image reconstruction in any plane (multiplanar reformatting [MPR])

  allows volume and surface rendering

1.121413

Inversion recovery technique

- basics

  180°–90°–180° RF pulsing

  initial 180° pulse inverts longitudinal magnetization (different from spin-echo technique)—longer time required for full T_1 recovery, thus greater T_1 contrast achieved

  TI (inversion time) = time between 180° and 90° pulses—chosen in range of T_1s of tissues being imaged to maximize T_1 contrast (150–450 msec)

    short TI—most signals are negative (not sufficient time for inverted magnetization to recover)

      absolute (magnitude) reconstruction—converts negative signals to positive, reversing apparent tissue contrast; can lead to reduced contrast between tissues and boundary artifacts if some tissues have recovered past zero

      phase sensitive reconstruction—maintains correct tissue magnitudes

    null ("bounce") point

      since magnetization is inverted, it must cross through a null point (zero) upon recovery

      TI can be chosen so that signal from a specific tissue (such as fat) has zero longitudinal magnetization (is crossing from negative to positive), with suppression of such tissue

  TE—short (<30 msec) to minimize T_2 contrast

  TR—long (>2000 msec) to allow full longitudinal recovery (thus long scan times)

- contrast dependency

  heavy T_1-weighting

- utility

  fat suppression (choice of TI to null signal from fat)—orbital imaging

  anatomic detail

1.121414

Fat suppression techniques

- utility

  improved visualization of structures otherwise obscured by fat—for example contents of orbit improved visualization of contrast enhancement in areas which contain large amounts of fat—for example the neck

Spectral (= frequency selective) saturation = CHESS (chemical shift selective saturation)

- basics

    fat and water separated on basis of differences in Larmor frequencies (resonant frequencies of protons in lipids and in water are separated by 3.5 ppm)

    frequency selective saturation pulse is applied prior to imaging pulses

- advantages

    can be applied to any imaging technique

    yields effective fat suppression (in small field-of-view)

    does not increase imaging time

- disadvantages

    difficult to achieve uniform fat suppression in all dimensions (requires high main field homogeneity throughout imaging volume)

Short tau inversion recovery (STIR)

- good fat suppression with correct choice of TI (which is field strength dependent)
- long scan times

1.121417

Magnetization transfer

- basics

    an intrinsic tissue characteristic (like T_1, T_2, and spin density)

    two hydrogen pools exist, one restricted (protons bound to complex molecular structures) and one freely mobile (water)

    freely mobile pool is that which is typically imaged (routine MR studies), due to extremely short T_2 of restricted pool

    restricted pool can be selectively saturated (by RF excitation), with transfer of magnetization to freely mobile pool

    result—shortening of T_1 of freely mobile pool and lower overall signal (since this pool is also partially saturated)

- utility

    improved vessel contrast in magnetic resonance angiography (MRA)

    improved visualization of intravenous (IV) contrast (gadolinium [Gd] chelate) on T_1-spin-echo scans

---

1.12142

Magnetic resonance angiography (MRA)

- two distinct imaging techniques

    time-of-flight (TOF)—detects signal amplitude difference between stationary and moving tissue phase contrast—detects signal phase difference between stationary and moving tissue

- image reconstruction

    maximum intensity projection (MIP)—most common method to postprocess MRA data for visual display

        voxels of high intensity from entire 3-D data set are displayed as if viewed from a given perspective

Two-dimensional time-of-flight (2-D TOF) MRA

- basics

    blood flow into imaging volume enhances vessel SI relative to background

    GRE techniques are employed, with gradient moment nulling (to minimize motion artifacts)

        by use of short TR, stationary tissue signal is saturated (suppressed), but fresh unsaturated blood flowing into slice has not been exposed to RF and thus is high SI

        vessel contrast dependent on:

            1. physiologic parameters (velocity, directionality, transit time in slice)
            2. measurement parameters (flip angle, slice thickness, slice orientation, TR)
            3. relaxation parameters (T_1, T_2)

    can void selectively arterial or venous flow, when flow is parallel (as in neck)—by use of saturation pulses

- advantages (vs. 3-D)

    fast—for limited number of slices

    improved slow flow detection

    improved background suppression

- disadvantages (vs. 3-D)

    signal is lost (saturated) from vessels which course within a slice (lie in plane)

    poor resolution in slice direction (typically 1.5–3 mm), with MIP reconstruction thus poor

    slices obtained sequentially in time, with patient motion leading to artifactual vessel discontinuity

Three-dimensional time-of-flight (3-D TOF) MRA

- basics

    technique of choice for visualization of intracranial arterial vasculature

    moderate background tissue suppression

    thick slab of tissue excited (vs. individual slices, as in 2-D TOF MRA), with this dimension phase encoded

    high resolution in all three dimensions

    effect of flip angle—higher vessel contrast, but poorer depth penetration (visualization of a vessel as it courses deep into imaging volume) with high flip angles

TOF disadvantages (both 2-D and 3-D)

- loss of vessel visualization with turbulent flow
- overestimation of vessel stenoses

Phase-contrast MRA

- basics

  good visualization of major vascular structures, with velocity and directionality information

  to depict flow in all three directions, four data sets must be acquired (one velocity encoded in each axis, and one as a reference)
- advantages (vs. TOF)

  provides quantitative information regarding velocity and direction of flow

  superior background suppression
- disadvantages (vs. TOF)

  long scan time

  accentuated pulsation artifacts

  cannot isolate venous and arterial flow

1.12143

Perfusion imaging

- rapid imaging with observation of first-pass effect of contrast agent bolus through tissue
- most methods observe negative enhancement (T_2 and T_2^*) effect of contrast agent, whether a gadolinium (Gd) or dysprosium (Dy) chelate is used
- information typically obtained is qualitative—quantitation of regional cerebral blood volume (rCBV) requires evaluation of concentration-time curve

---

1.12144

Diffusion imaging

- basics

  modification of imaging technique, by use of extremely strong gradient fields, to increase sensitivity to molecular motion

    motion on molecular level then causes a reduction in observed signal amplitude

    tissues can be differentiated on basis of change in signal amplitude when scans with diffusion and without diffusion weighting are compared

    tissue diffusion coefficients can be calculated
- utility

  visualization of cytotoxic edema (early infarction)

  evaluation of myelinization

diffusion information is directionally dependent (application of sensitizing gradient is made along single axis)

1.121419

SNR (signal-to-noise ratio) and CNR (contrast-to-noise ratio)

- for good tissue differentiation (CNR), there must be high SNR and intrinsic contrast between tissues

    lower contrast between tissues requires increased SNR to maintain CNR

- high SNR typically requires long scan times

$$\text{SNR} \approx \frac{(\text{FOVread})(\text{FOVphase})\text{Wslice}(\text{NavTs})^{1/2}}{\text{Nread}(\text{Nphase})^{1/2}}$$

where:

    FOVread = field-of-view in the readout direction
    FOVphase = field-of-view in the phase-encoding direction
    Wslice = slice thickness
    Nav = number of averages or data acquisitions = NEX
    Ts = time to measure each MR signal (bandwidth = Nread/Ts)
    Nread = number of measurements of each MR signal (readout steps)
    Nphase = number of phase-encoding steps

to note:

    (FOVread)/Nread = voxel dimension in readout direction = Δx
    (FOVphase)/Nphase = voxel dimension in phase-encoding direction = Δy
    Wslice = voxel dimension in slice select direction = Δz
    1/Ts = bandwidth in units of Hz/pixel

scan time
(for spin-echo technique) = (TR)(Nav)(Nphase)

incorporating above, equation becomes:

$$\text{SNR} = (\Delta x)(\Delta y)(\Delta z)(\text{NavTsNphase})^{1/2}$$

Common ways to influence SNR

Parameter	Action	Increase in SNR
FOV (read & phase)	double it	4 times
Slice thickness	double it	2 times
Averages	double it	1.4 times
Bandwidth	half it	1.4 times

Of above techniques, only changing averages affects scan time (doubling averages—increases SNR by factor of 1.4, but doubles scan time)

thick sections—suffer from partial volume effects and loss of detail

thin sections (pituitary, IAC studies)—require increase in averages to achieve acceptable SNR

high spatial resolution (using small FOV)—achieved only at substantial cost in SNR (halving FOV reduces SNR by factor of four) wraparound (aliasing) of tissue structures in phase-encoding direction occurs if FOV is smaller than object imaged (potential pitfall)

use of oversampling (extended matrix) in readout direction eliminates wraparound in this axis at no cost in scan time or SNR

- high spatial resolution (using large acquisition matrix, for example 512 × 512)—achieved only at substantial cost in SNR

more prominent truncation artifacts with smaller matrix size

increased scan time with larger matrix size

Slice profile (2-D imaging)

- in practice, excitation of slice of tissue with distinct edges (like "slice of bread") not possible in MR

excitation of tissue, with reduced flip angle, well beyond desired slice border is typical

- slice-to-slice interference ("cross-talk")—leads to loss of image contrast and SNR

minimized by use of small gaps between slices (typically 10–30% of slice thickness)

Partial data methods

- not all of k-space is sampled (half-Fourier technique = half of k-space sampled)
- scan time is reduced proportionate with number of phase-encoding steps
- SNR is reduced
- spatial resolution is unchanged

Asymmetrical FOV

- reduction of FOV in phase-encoding direction, accompanied by reduction in number of phase-encoding steps
- scan time is reduced
- SNR is reduced
- spatial resolution is unchanged (typically)
- potential artifacts from wraparound

Artifacts

- magnetic susceptibility

definition—degree to which a material becomes magnetized

different tissues have different magnetic susceptibilities

spin-echo technique—180° pulse compensates for field errors, with little effect of magnetic susceptibility

GRE technique

signal loss noted between regions with different susceptibility

largest susceptibility effect seen at air-tissue interfaces

increasing TE increases susceptibility artifacts

lower sampling bandwidth increases susceptibility artifacts

- metal artifact
    - metal distorts main magnetic field, with result:
        - signal loss
        - local image distortion
    - worse with:
        - GRE (vs. spin-echo) technique
        - longer TE
        - lower bandwidth
        - lower spatial resolution
- chemical shift artifact
    - basis—slight difference in Larmor resonance frequency between fat and water
    - result—pixel misregistration in frequency-encoding direction, seen as high or low signal intensity line at interface between fat and water
        - accentuated by:
            - higher main magnetic field (1.5 T)
            - use of low bandwidth pulse sequences
                - low bandwidth typically not used with T_1 sequences, due to high SI of fat and prominent chemical shift artifact
                - low bandwidth commonly employed with T_2 (long TE) sequences, due to lower SI of fat and less apparent chemical shift artifact
- motion artifact
    - basis—gross patient motion, vessel pulsation, and CSF pulsation
        - SI of moving structures is mismapped spatially
    - result—artifactual ghosts in phase-encoding direction (regardless of direction of motion); can add destructively (giving signal voids) or constructively (giving artifactual high SI)
    - compensation schemes
        - gradient moment nulling (= MAST [motion artifact suppression technique] = "motion compensation")
            - additional gradient pulses added to compensate for phase errors
                - compensation can be first (velocity), second (acceleration), or third (jerk) order in degree
                - compensation can be along one, two, or three axes (frequency and slice select directions are most important)
            - commonly used clinically (first order correction, one or two axes)
            - implementation prolongs minimum TE which can be achieved
        - spatial presaturation (= "sat" pulse)
            - application of spatially selective RF pulse to saturate spins in certain region (suppressing SI from this region)
                - increases specific absorption rate (SAR)—potential problem with heat deposition

reduces number of slices which can be performed with multislice technique (application of sat pulse requires time within pulse sequence, which otherwise could be used to acquire additional slices)

"through-plane" (perpendicular to slice orientation)—not commonly employed in head imaging, but often used in spine imaging to eliminate SI from anterior soft tissues and thus diminish motion artifacts

"in-plane" (parallel-to-slice orientation)—commonly employed above and below imaging volume to eliminate SI from inflowing blood and thus diminish pulsation artifacts

- aliasing (= "wraparound")

    basis—signal is spatially encoded by frequency and phase information, with tissue outside intended FOV not uniquely coded

    more likely to occur with small FOV

    result—image wraparound (can occur in phase-encoding or readout direction), with signal from outside FOV superimposed on image

    compensation techniques

    readout direction—oversampling, with no cost in time or SNR

    phase-encoding direction—oversampling, which adds imaging time

    use of spatial presaturation

    use of surface coil

- data truncation

    basis—finite sampling of MR signal (number of data samples), with artifact introduced by Fourier transformation

    result—ringing ("Gibbs") artifact (parallel-to-high-contrast tissue interfaces, dying away at distance) and loss of edge definition

    compensation techniques

    filtering (which can also induce blurring)

    acquisition of image with higher spatial resolution

Safety issues—MR

- risks associated with metal implants

    movement/dislodgement

    electrical current induction/conduction

    heating

    image artifacts (nondiagnostic scan)

- specific implants/materials

    intracranial aneurysm clip—ferromagnetic clips can experience substantial deflection, with potential to dislodge, and are contraindication to MR scan

    electrically, mechanically, or magnetically activated implants are contraindication to MR scan—these include pacemakers, defibrillators (implanted), neurostimulators, bone-growth stimulators, cochlear implants, drug-infusion pumps (implanted)

    intracardiac wires are major concern due to potential for current induction (with fibrillation or thermal injury)—these include temporary pacing wires, external pacing wires, Swan-Ganz catheters other contraindicated metal implants/objects—vascular clamps (some types), heart valves (some types), ferromagnetic intravascular coils (filters, stents), ocular implants (some types), McGee stapedectomy piston prosthesis, ferromagnetic fragments (pellets, shrapnel, bullets)—when located in vital areas (specifically globe) or near nerves or blood vessels, Dacomed Omniphase penile implant

- external objects of potential risk

gating leads, halo vests, physiologic monitoring equipment—can cause tissue burns, unless MR compatible

ferromagnetic objects—can act as projectiles

- pregnancy

safety of imaging for fetus not established

Normal Anatomy (and Definitions) ....

Normal intracranial anatomy

- structural

frontal lobe demarcated posteriorly from parietal lobe by central sulcus, and inferiorly from temporal lobe by lateral sulcus (sylvian fissure)

parietal lobe demarcated from occipital lobe by parieto-occipital sulcus, and inferiorly from temporal lobe by lateral sulcus (and its imaginary linear continuation posteriorly)

- functional

primary motor area (Brodmann area 4)—precentral gyrus

primary somatesthetic (body's sensations) area (Brodmann areas 1, 2, and 3)—postcentral gyrus

Arterial vascular territories

- anterior cerebral artery (ACA)

supplies anterior two-thirds of medial cerebral surface and 1 cm of superomedial brain over convexity

recurrent artery of Heubner (originates from A1 or A2 segment)—supplies caudate head, anterior limb of internal capsule, part of putamen

anterior choroidal artery (arises from supraclinoid internal carotid artery)—supplies posterior limb of internal capsule, portions of thalamus, caudate, globus pallidus, cerebral peduncle

- middle cerebral artery (MCA)

supplies lateral cerebrum, insula, and anterior and lateral temporal lobes

lenticulostriate arteries (originate from M1 segment)—supply basal ganglia, anterior limb of internal capsule

"sylvian triangle"—MCA branches that loop over insula deep in sylvian fissure

- posterior cerebral artery (PCA)

supplies occipital lobe and medial temporal lobe

thalamoperforating arteries (arise from P1 and posterior communicating artery)—supply medial ventral thalamus, posterior limb of internal capsule

- posterior inferior cerebellar artery (PICA)—supplies tonsil, inferior vermis and cerebellum
- anterior inferior cerebellar artery (AICA)—supplies anterior cerebellar hemisphere
- superior cerebellar artery (SCA)—supplies superior cerebellar hemisphere

Vascular shifts (arteriography)

- anterior cerebral artery (all seen on anteroposterior view)
    round shift—ACA shifted across midline by deep frontal mass
    square shift—ACA shifted across midline by temporal mass
    proximal shift—proximal ACA shifted across midline by anterioinferior mass
    distal shift—distal ACA shifted across midline (sharp angle at falx) by posterior mass

Brain herniations (acquired)

- subfalcine
- transtentorial (descending much more common than ascending)
- tonsillar
- sphenoid ridge (ascending or descending)

Pituitary gland

- general information
    adenohyphophysis = anterior pituitary
    neurohypophysis = posterior pituitary
- shape/measurements/imaging characteristics
    upward convexity (but <10 mm height)—normal in young women
    demonstrates intense enhancement following IV-contrast administration, due to lack of blood-brain barrier
    MR
        posterior pituitary is hyperintense (like fat) on T_1 scans in more than 50% of patients
        small low SI foci seen within pituitary on enhanced T_1 scans in 15% of asymptomatic individuals (correspond to small cysts)
- imaging
    thin sections (≤3 mm on MR, sagittal, and coronal) important for diagnostic evaluation

Internal auditory canal (IAC)

- anatomy
    bony foramen within petrous portion of temporal bone
    contains 7th (facial) and 8th (vestibulocochlear) nerve complex

7th nerve

lies in anterosuperior quadrant of IAC (in cross-section), runs to geniculate ganglion laterally

8th nerve

cochlear division lies in anteroinferior quadrant

superior and inferior vestibular nerves (supply information concerning equilibrium) lie in superior and inferior posterior quadrants

cochlea lies anterior (within inner ear)

vestibule lies posterior

semicircular canals—lateral (horizontal orientation), superior, and posterior

- imaging appearance

nerves—isointense to brain

cochlea, vestibule, semicircular canals, IAC (all contain fluid)—isointense to CSF

- imaging

thin sections (≤3 mm on MR, axial, and coronal) important for diagnostic evaluation

Normal myelination

- general information

begins in brainstem, progresses to cerebellum and cerebrum (order of myelination is central to peripheral, inferior to superior, and posterior to anterior)

T_1-weighted images—particularly useful to assess myelination in first 9 months of life

with normal myelination, white matter becomes higher SI (due to cholesterol, protein content)

T_2-weighted images—more useful to assess myelination after 6 months of age (however, longer TRs, 3000–4000 msec, are required for evaluation of brain under 2 years of age)

with normal myelination, white matter becomes lower SI (due to myelin becoming progressively hydrophobic—low-water content—as it matures)

- newborn

dorsal pons, superior and inferior cerebellar peduncles, posterior limb of internal capsule, and ventral lateral thalamus demonstrate partial myelination (decreased SI on T_2, increased SI on T_1)

corpus callosum—not myelinated, appears thin

- 6 months of age

T_1

cerebellum, posterior limb and genu of internal capsule, occipital lobe, posterior centrum semiovale—normally myelinated (high SI on T_1)

corpus callosum—still thin, but now partially myelinated (high SI on T_1)

T_2

> only posterior limb of internal capsule demonstrates low SI (indicative of myelination)

- 12 months of age

    T_1

    > adult pattern of myelination (deep and peripheral white matter)—this is reached by 9 months of age

    T_2

    > deep white matter (internal capsule, corpus callosum, corona radiata)—mature, with low SI

    > white matter of frontal, temporal, parietal, and occipital lobes and peripheral (subcortical) white matter—not mature, with SI isointense to gray matter

- 2 years of age

    T_2

    > deep and superficial white matter of frontal, temporal, parietal, and occipital lobes—low SI (like adult)

    >> SI may not be as low as internal capsule (this occurs by 3 years of age)

    > deep white matter of parietal lobes (surrounding ventricular trigones)—last to completely myelinate ("terminal myelinization")

    >> mild hyperintensity on T_2 may persist up to 10 years of age

---

1.123

Normal venous anatomy

- central venous anatomy—paired internal cerebral veins join basal vein of Rosenthal to form vein of Galen; vein of Galen is joined by inferior sagittal sinus (which lies within free edge of falx) to form straight sinus, which drains to torcular herophili
- superficial venous anatomy

    superficial cerebral veins join to form superior sagittal sinus midline, which drains to torcular herophili, with flow continuing via transverse sinuses (often quite asymmetric, with the right usually dominant) to sigmoid sinus, to jugular bulb, and then to internal jugular vein

    three, large, named superficial veins

    > superficial middle cerebral vein—lies in sylvian fissure, drains into cavernous or sphenoparietal sinus

    > vein of Trolard—joins superior sagittal sinus and superficial middle cerebral vein

    > vein of Labbé—joins transverse sinus and superficial middle cerebral vein

- imaging of venous system

    MR

    > best demonstrated on 2-D TOF MRA

    > improved depiction on spin-echo imaging following IV-contrast administration

1.124

Normal arterial anatomy

- circle of Willis
    - complete in 25% of population
    - variants (incomplete circle)
        - fetal origin of PCA (from internal carotid artery (ICA) instead of from basilar artery, 22%)—P1 segment usually also hypoplastic in this circumstance
        - posterior communicating artery hypoplastic—34%
        - anterior communicating artery hypoplastic—15%
        - A1 segment hypoplastic—10%
- external carotid artery
    - smaller of two terminal branches of common carotid artery
    - arises anterior and medial to ICA, then courses posterolaterally
    - major branches
        - superior thyroid artery
        - ascending pharyngeal artery
        - lingual artery
        - facial artery
        - occipital artery
        - posterior auricular artery
        - superficial temporal artery
        - internal maxillary artery
- internal carotid artery (ICA)
    - segments
        - cervical
        - petrous
        - cavernous (juxtasellar) [subsegments listed below]
            - ascending cavernous
            - genu
            - horizontal cavernous
            - anterior genu
        - intracranial (supraclinoid)
    - branches
        - meningohypophyseal trunk
        - ophthalmic artery
        - posterior communicating artery
- extracranial-intracranial vascular anastomoses
    - maxillary artery to ICA (via ethmoidal branches of maxillary artery to ethmoidal branches of ophthalmic to ICA)
    - occipital artery to vertebral artery
    - ascending pharyngeal artery to vertebral artery
    - ascending pharyngeal artery to ICA
    - facial artery (angular branch) to ICA (via ophthalmic)

- internal carotid-vertebral artery anastomoses (persistent embryonic circulatory patterns, listed cephalad to caudad)

  persistent trigeminal artery (most common)

  acoustic (otic) artery (very rare)

  hypoglossal artery

  proatlantal intersegmental artery

- pial-leptomeningeal anastomoses—additional potential source of collateral blood flow in occlusive vascular disease

---

1.127

Contrast media

- MR—for conventional brain and spine imaging, effect of contrast is visualized on T_1-weighted imaging and is seen as increase in SI (pre- and postcontrast T_1-weighted scans recommended, for definitive identification of contrast enhancement—otherwise other high SI materials such as blood and fat could be mistaken for contrast agent)

  type of agent—gadolinium (Gd) chelate

  Gd—a paramagnetic metal ion, the "active ingredient"

  chelate—tightly binds Gd ion and assures complete elimination by kidneys

  dose

  0.1 mmol/kg (0.2 cc/kg)—conventional

  0.3 mmol/kg—improved visualization of brain metastases and poorly enhancing lesions

  normal-enhancing structures—choroid plexus, pituitary, mucosal surfaces (especially nasal)

  principles of enhancement

  intra-axial lesions—enhancement seen with disruption of the blood-brain barrier

  extra-axial lesions—enhancement seen due to intrinsic vascularity

Normal Variants ....

1.134

Physiologic calcification

- general information

  glomus portion of choroid plexus (contained in atria of lateral ventricles)—most frequent portion of choroid plexus to calcify

  calcification usually globular and bilateral

  falx—increased density (calcification or ossification)—seen by computed tomography (CT) in up to 42% of adults

  typically an incidental finding

  higher incidence in hyper- and hypoparathyroidism, hypervitaminosis A and D

  due to normal low SI of falx on MR, calcification not commonly visualized, while ossification is well seen (due to high SI of fat within)

- imaging appearance
  CT—high attenuation
  MR
  T_1—variable appearance—low, intermediate, or increased SI (latter due to fatty matrix, or particulate calcium)
  T_2—low SI
  can demonstrate chemical shift artifact (due to fatty matrix within calcification)—in frequency-encoding direction

---

1.135

Variations in ventricular system

Cavum septum pellucidum

- general information
  septum pellucidum
  thin translucent plate, consisting of two laminae (leaves), lying in midline between frontal horns of lateral ventricles
  links hippocampus to hypothalamus (abnormalities of septum may have associated subtle neuropsychiatric symptoms)
  cavum septum pellucidum
  normal embryologic space
  seen in 100% of fetuses and premature infants
  seen in only 15% of infants by age 3–6 months
  can persist into adulthood—normal variant
  when large (>1 cm diameter)—can cause obstruction to CSF flow at foramen of Monro

Cavum septum vergae

- general information
  a normal embryologic cavity, like cavum septum pellucidum
  essentially a posterior extension of cavum septum pellucidum
  that portion of midline cavity posterior to columns of fornix, which ends (in midline) at splenium of corpus callosum
  begins to disappear at 6 months gestation
  when present in adult—normal variant
- imaging appearance
  midline CSF cavity, flash-shaped on axial images, directly posterior to cavum septum pellucidum

Cavum velum interpositum

- general information
  less common than cavum septum pellucidum or vergae
  defined by separation of crura of fornix between thalami and above third ventricle

cavum vergae lies superior to internal cerebral veins, which lie within a cavum velum interpositum

Absent septum pellucidum

- general information

  rare anomaly, almost always signifies major neurologic disease

  associated with holoprosencephaly, septo-optic dysplasia, agenesis of corpus callosum, schizencephaly, basilar encephaloceles, hydranencephaly, Chiari II malformation

  can be acquired, due to severe chronic hydrocephalus (with rupture and disintegration of septum)

  due to absence of septum, fornix lies in abnormally low position, with horizontal orientation

1.136

Dilated perivascular spaces

- general information

  perivascular space = Virchow-Robin space—a normal CSF space, surrounding perforating arteries entering brain, represents invagination of subarachnoid space

  dilated perivascular spaces—common locations

  inferior third of basal ganglia (usually <5 mm diameter, but can be larger), adjacent to anterior commissure, following course of lenticulostriate arteries

  differentiation from lacunar infarcts—latter are more ovoid (slitlike), occur in upper two-thirds of basal ganglia, and do not have CSF SI on all MR pulse sequences (hyperintense to CSF on scans with intermediate T_2-weighting)

  high convexity white matter of centrum semiovale (<2 mm diameter), following course of nutrient arteries

  midbrain (<1.5 mm diameter), junction of substantia nigra and cerebral peduncle, following branches of collicular arteries

- imaging appearance

  commonly noted on MR, rarely visualized on CT

Congenital Anomaly, Developmental Abnormality ...

1.1412

Holoprosencephaly

- general information

  congenital malformation of brain, characterized by failure of cleavage and differentiation in forebrain

  divided into three subcategories, listed in order of decreasing severity (division is artificial, variants represent a spectrum of disease)—septum pellucidum absent in all alobar—thalami fused, third ventricle absent, falx absent (no interhemispheric fissure); single crescent-shaped ventricle connected to large dorsal cyst; rarely imaged—infants stillborn or of short lifespan

semilobar—interhemispheric fissure and falx present posteriorly, with partial separation of thalami by small third ventricle, rudimentary temporal horn, splenium of corpus callosum present

lobar—falx and interhemispheric fissure extend into frontal region, anterior falx dysplastic, frontal horns of abnormal configuration, frontal lobes may be hypoplastic

clinical presentation—microcephaly, seizures, developmental delay

in more severe forms, may be hypotelorism and a midline facial cleft

- imaging appearance

coronal scans (MR) useful to demonstrate frontal lobe abnormalities

---

1.1413

Agenesis of the corpus callosum

- general information

largest interhemispheric commissure in brain

development in fetus—between 8th and 20th weeks, in anterior to posterior fashion (genu first, then body, then splenium), with exception of rostrum which forms last

primary dysgenesis—caused by insult during development, with total agenesis due to early insult, and partial agenesis to later insult

axons that normally cross midline instead run along medial borders of lateral ventricles (parallel to interhemispheric fissure), forming bundles of Probst

associated with other anomalies of brain in 80%—Chiari II, Dandy-Walker, interhemispheric cysts, neuronal migration anomalies, basilar encephaloceles

callosal abnormality best imaged in sagittal plane

- imaging appearance (in addition to callosal abnormality)

wide separation and parallel orientation of lateral ventricles

crescentic shape of lateral ventricles (in particular, frontal horns) on coronal images ("devil's horns")

superior extension of third ventricle between lateral ventricles

dilatation of trigones and occipital horns (colpocephaly)

radial orientation of mesial hemispheric gyri

1.1419

Neuronal migrational abnormalities—neurons of cerebral cortex arise in fetus in germinal matrix along lateral ventricles, major neuron migration to final position in peripheral cortex occurs during 8–16 weeks of development

Pachygyria

- general information

  terminology

  pachygyria, agyria, and lissencephaly describe spectrum of involvement characterized by a simplified gyral pattern (broad thick gyri, fewer than normal in number)

  agyria = lissencephaly—most severe form, brain resembles immature fetus with few rudimentary gyri (divided by primary sulci and fissures)

  pachygyria ("pachy" = thick)—least severe form, more completely developed gyri, most commonly diffuse, with relative sparing of temporal lobes (but can be focal and unilateral)

  associated conditions—agenesis of corpus callosum, heterotopic gray matter

  clinical presentation—microcephaly, seizures, mental retardation, developmental delay

- imaging appearance

  MR superior to CT for demonstration of abnormal convolutional pattern and thickened cortex

  often a circumferential band of high SI on T_2 within cortex, corresponding to cell sparse layer

  coronal images best demonstrate relative sparing of temporal lobes

Polymicrogyria

- general information

  multiple abnormal tiny indentations along brain surface (gross appearance), thickened cortex, abnormal cortical histology (four layers vs. normal six), decreased white matter

  can be unilateral, often in MCA distribution

- imaging appearance—MR

  decreased number of broad, thick, smooth gyri (indentations of cortex too small to be seen)

  often with associated anomalous venous drainage, large draining vein in deep sulcus

  difficult to differentiate from pachygyria (which is less common, and usually bilateral)

Schizencephaly

- general information

  characterized by presence of gray matter-lined cleft

  cleft extends from cortex to ventricles

  unilateral or bilateral

  spectrum of appearance, in terms of separation of gray matter-lined walls

  fusion (fused lips, closed gap)

  wide separation (wide gap)

pathogenesis—episode of hypotension in utero, with subsequent infarction in watershed area (germinal matrix along lateral ventricle)

associated abnormalities—pachygyria, polymicrogyria, heterotopic gray matter

schizencephaly and septo-optic dysplasia are frequently found together, both conditions are associated with absent septum pellucidum

clinical presentation—intractable seizures, motor dysfunction (weakness to paralysis), developmental delay

neurologic disability ranges from mild to severe

- imaging appearance

MR—superior to CT for detection of gray matter-lined cleft and associated abnormalities

- differential diagnosis

porencephaly—abnormal CSF space, due to destruction of brain, which can communicate with ventricle but is not lined by gray matter

Heterotopic gray matter

- general information

displaced masses of nerve cells (gray matter)

found anywhere from embryologic site of development (periventricular) to final destination after cell migration (cortex)

type of involvement

most common form—small nests adjacent to lateral ventricles ("nodular")

when focal, often near anterior and posterior horns, with projection into ventricular system as small nodules

laminar—large areas of involvement, in white matter regions

clinical presentation—seizures; when isolated (without other congenital abnormalities)—late onset, mild symptoms

- imaging appearance

MR—isointense with gray matter on all pulse sequences

- differential diagnosis

subependymal nodules in tuberous sclerosis—these have associated calcification, with cortical involvement in tuberous sclerosis an additional differentiating feature

---

1.1423

Porencephaly

- general information

focal cavity due to brain destruction (vascular accident) during third trimester of fetal life (strict definition)

term has been used indiscriminately to include any non-neoplastic cavity within brain, with etiologies including vascular insult, trauma, infection, and surgery

immature brain does not mount glial reaction, thus necrotic tissue is completely resorbed without formation of surrounding gliosis

neuronal migration is complete by third trimester, thus not associated with migrational abnormalities

may or may not communicate with ventricle or subarachnoid space (often abuts ventricle, with intervening intact ependyma)

- imaging appearance—well-demarcated cavity filled with CSF

CT—low density

MR—isointense with CSF on all pulse sequences

1.1452

Dandy-Walker complex—term which includes Dandy-Walker malformation, Dandy-Walker variant, and mega cisterna magna; suggested on basis that these three entities may represent a disease continuum (posterior fossa developmental anomalies)

Dandy-Walker malformation

- general information

defined by presence of three features:

high position of tentorium

dysgenesis/agenesis of vermis

cystic dilatation of fourth ventricle (which bulges posteriorly, frequently occupying much of posterior fossa)

additional commonly associated features

hypoplasia of cerebellar hemispheres

scalloping of inner table of occipital bone

associated abnormalities

hydrocephalus (75%)

dysgenesis of corpus callosum (25%)

heterotopic gray matter (10%)

pathogenesis (theory)—delayed opening or obstruction of foramen of Magendie

- imaging appearance

MR—imaging in sagittal plane essential for definition of structural abnormalities (in congenital abnormalities of the brain, imaging in all three perpendicular planes is recommended)

Dandy-Walker variant

- dysgenesis of vermis and cystic dilatation of fourth ventricle, but without enlargement of posterior fossa

Mega cisterna magna

- enlarged CSF space (large cisterna magna) posterior to cerebellum, with normal cerebellum (vermis and fourth ventricle), without mass effect

- by MR or CT without intrathecal contrast, cannot be differentiated from arachnoid cyst that does not have mass effect

1.1466

Retrocerebellar (posterior fossa) arachnoid cyst

- general information

    collection of CSF in retrocerebellar location not communicating directing with fourth ventricle

        like all arachnoid cysts, has a discrete membrane, which is usually not seen on imaging

    most common in midline (retrovermian)

    size of posterior fossa, position of tentorium and straight sinus, and cerebellar vermis and hemispheres are normal

    clinical presentation—most asymptomatic (incidental imaging finding), rarely ataxia due to compression of cerebellum

- imaging appearance

    MR

        CSF SI on all pulse sequences

        can have:

            mass effect on cerebellum

            scalloping of inner table of calvaria

1.1473

Chiari I malformation

- general information

    congenital displacement (>2 mm below posterior lip of foramen magnum) of cerebellar tonsils into cervical canal (tonsillar herniation)

        two-thirds have herniation below C1

    clinical presentation—usually asymptomatic; when symptomatic, patients present with cerebellar signs (ataxia, nystagmus), or symptoms of cranial nerve/brainstem compression

- imaging appearance—MR

    pointed or wedge-shaped cerebellar tonsils (on sagittal imaging)

    fourth ventricle in normal position

    may be accompanying o bliteration of cisterna magna, and downward displacement of inferior vermis

    associated conditions

        syringohydromyelia

        hydrocephalus

        craniocervical junction anomalies (occipitalization of C1, Klippel-Feil syndrome, basilar impression)

Chiari II malformation

- general information

    complex congenital brain anomaly—hindbrain dysgenesis with inferior displacement and elongation of brainstem, tonsils, vermis, and fourth ventricle

    associated with myelomeningocele in close to 100%

- imaging appearance
    - features (not all need to be present)
        - infratentorial/spine
            - small posterior fossa, low insertion of tentorium—which is dysplastic with widened incisura allowing cerebellum to extend superiorly ("towering cerebellum")
            - cerebellar dysplasia (abnormal orientation of folia, extension of hemispheres anteriorly to surround brainstem)
            - elongated, inferiorly displaced fourth ventricle (ballooned in 10%)
            - widened foramen magnum
            - cervicomedullary kinking (due to inferior displacement of medulla)
            - cervical syrinx
        - supratentorial
            - obstructive hydrocephalus (98%)
            - callosal dysgenesis (75%)
            - fusion of colliculi ("tectal beaking," 60%)
            - anteroinferior pointing of frontal horns
            - absent septum pellucidum
            - large massa intermedia
            - hypoplasia/fenestration of falx, with interdigitation of cerebral gyri
            - stenogyria (multiple, small closely spaced gyri with normal cortex histologically)
            - abnormal CSF spaces (especially interhemispheric) after shunting

Chiari III malformation

Chiari II malformation with low occipital or high cervical encephalocele (very rare)

1.1475

Basilar invagination ("impression")

- general information
    - bony craniovertebral junction abnormality—odontoid high in position relative to foramen magnum, specifically >5 mm above Chamberlain's line—which extends from posterior edge of hard palate to posterior edge of foramen magnum
    - dens can compress or displace medulla
    - etiology
        - due to primary bone anomaly (often associated with assimilation of posterior arch of C1 to occiput)
        - secondary to other primary disease—osteoporosis, osteomalacia, Paget's disease, fibrous dysplasia, achondroplasia, osteogenesis imperfecta

platybasia may also be present (flattened relationship between anterior and middle cranial fossae, with angle formed >140°)

clinical presentation—headache, neurologic deficits, symptoms from vertebrobasilar artery compression

- imaging appearance

plain film—adequate to assess bony abnormalities

MR—used to assess anatomic distortion of brainstem/cord

1.15

Septo-optic dysplasia

- general information

congenital anomaly with abnormal septum pellucidum (mild dysplasia to complete absence) and hypoplasia of optic nerves

50% also have schizencephaly

clinical presentation—varied (septo-optic dysplasia is not a single homogeneous entity)—blindness, seizures, hypothalamic-pituitary dysfunction, developmental delay, growth retardation

1.181

Lysosomal storage diseases (congenital enzyme deficiencies)—subtypes:

1. sphingolipidoses (includes gangliosidoses [Tay-Sachs], Krabbe, Fabry, Gaucher, Niemann-Pick, and Farber)
2. mucopolysaccharidoses (includes Hurler, Hunter, Sanfilippo, Morquio, Scheie, and Maroteaux-Lamy)—all display coarse facial features ("gargoylism"), with skeletal and multiple organ involvement
3. mucolipidoses
4. oligosaccharidoses
5. glycogenoses

Hurler's disease—most common form of mucopolysaccharidoses (type I)

- defect in enzyme α-ʟ-iduronidase
- clinical presentation—mental retardation, deafness, short stature, corneal clouding, coarse facial features, death by teen years
- imaging appearance—ventriculomegaly, cerebral atrophy, J-shaped sella; MR—cavitated white matter lesions, diffuse white matter T_2 hyperintensity (gliosis, demyelination)

Hunter's disease—second most common form of mucopolysaccharidoses (type II)

- imaging appearance (as with all mucopolysaccharidoses)—cerebral atrophy, prominent perivascular spaces

1.1831

Neurofibromatosis—autosomal dominant disease, with two distinct syndromes described

Neurofibromatosis type 1

- general information

  = von Recklinghausen's disease

  more common form (20 times that of type 2)

  abnormality localized to chromosome 17

  characterized by café au lait spots (on skin), axillary freckles, iris hamartomas, multiple subcutaneous nodules (peripheral nerve tumors), tumors of head (optic nerve gliomas, which can be bilateral, and brain gliomas) and spinal canal

- imaging appearance—MR

  high T_2 SI abnormalities (likely hamartomas) in globus pallidus, brainstem, and cerebellar white matter—without mass effect or abnormal enhancement

  > lesions of globus pallidus can be slightly hyperintense on T_1

Neurofibromatosis type 2

- general information

  characterized by bilateral acoustic neuromas

  other common neoplasms—cranial and spinal meningiomas, cranial nerve tumors, paraspinal neurofibromas, spinal cord ependymomas

  abnormality localized to chromosome 22

  can also have café au lait spots, subcutaneous nodules

1.1832

Tuberous sclerosis

- general information

  one of the neurocutaneous syndromes, with autosomal dominant inheritance (mutation of chromosome 9)

  cutaneous lesions include leaf-shaped hypopigmented spots (trunk and limbs), adenoma sebaceum (small pink spots scattered over face in butterfly pattern), rough, thickened yellow skin over lumbosacral region (shagreen patch)

  mental retardation and infantile epilepsy—common

  brain tumors in 2%; most common lesion—subependymal giant cell astrocytoma (classic location within lateral ventricular wall, with obstructive hydrocephalus due to blockage of foramen of Monro)

- imaging appearance

  CT

  > calcified subependymal nodules
  >
  > peripheral calcifications
  >
  > parenchymal hypointensity
  >
  > ventricular dilatation (due to atrophy)

  MR

  > subependymal nodules—best seen on T_1

multiple parenchymal lesions (tubers = hamartomas)—best seen on T_2 (high SI)

involve cortical and subcortical regions, gray and white matter

"gyral core"—abnormality confined to subcortical white matter core of an expanded gyrus

"sulcal island"—involvement of two adjacent gyri, with sparing of normal intervening cortex lining the sulcus

1.1833

Sturge-Weber syndrome (encephalotrigeminal angiomatosis)

- general information

rare nonfamilial neurocutaneous syndrome

characteristic lesions include: port-wine stain, leptomeningeal angiomatosis (usually ipsilateral to facial nevus), cerebral atrophy, buphthalmos (congenital-enlarged globe and glaucoma), choroidal angioma, seizures, mental retardation, hemiparesis, hemiatrophy

pathogenesis (intracranial lesion)—lack of superficial cortical veins (may be enlarged deep veins), with tissue hypoxia (chronic) and cortical atrophy

- imaging appearance

CT—focal curvilinear calcifications with atrophy of adjacent cerebral cortex

MR—focal leptomeningeal enhancement with cortical atrophy

Inflammation ....

1.206

Human immunodeficiency virus (HIV) encephalitis

- general information

direct neurotrophic effect of virus

- imaging appearance

diffuse periventricular white matter T_2 high SI

Progressive multifocal leukoencephalopathy (PML)

- general information

viral demyelinating disease

seen in immunocompromised patients, particularly acquired immunodeficiency syndrome (AIDS)

rapid disease progression, with death in 6 months

- imaging appearance

MR—focal areas of abnormal white matter with high SI on T_2, often in an asymmetrical distribution

1.2074

Toxoplasmosis

- general information
  - ubiquitous obligate intracellular protozoan
  - causes mild self-limited infection with mild lymphadenopathy and fever in normal adult
  - approximately 50% of US population has been exposed and has antibodies
  - mode of transmission—insufficiently cooked meat, cat feces
  - important pathogen in fetus and immunocompromised patient
    - transmitted to fetus during acute infection of mother—with result being diffuse/focal encephalitis
    - the most common intracranial opportunistic infection in AIDS—with reactivation of latent infection or fulminant acquired infection
      - treatment—pyrimethamine and sulfadiazine
- imaging appearance
  - congenital toxoplasmosis
    - scattered intracranial calcifications throughout brain (vs. congenital infection with cytomegalovirus which demonstrates predominantly periventricular calcifications)
    - atrophy
  - immunocompromised patient (AIDS)
    - focal region of high SI on T_2 (lesion itself), often with surrounding edema
    - nodular or ring enhancement
    - location in basal ganglia or cerebral hemisphere (gray-white matter junction)
- differential diagnosis—multiple ring-enhancing lesions in the immunocompromised patient
  - lymphoma
  - metastatic disease

1.2083

Neurocysticercosis

- general information
  - infection of the central nervous system (CNS) by larval stage of pork tapeworm *(Taenia solium)*
    - viable larvae survive 4–5 years, with pronounced host inflammatory reaction on parasite death
  - clinical presentation—seizures (parenchymal cysts), obstructive hydrocephalus (intraventricular cysts)
  - treatment—praziquantel (an oral anthelmintic agent)

- imaging appearance

    CT—parenchymal calcifications, at gray-white matter junction; intraventricular cysts difficult to identify

    MR—small cysts, isointense to CSF on T_1 and T_2, with surrounding high T_2 SI (edema), ring enhancement (cyst wall) postcontrast

- differential diagnosis—small ring-enhancing lesion

    metastasis

    brain abscess

1.22

Neurosarcoidosis

- general information

    two main patterns of brain involvement

        focal or diffuse granulomatous leptomeningitis involving skull base

            clinical presentation—cranial nerve palsies, meningeal signs, hypothalamic dysfunction

        parenchymal involvement by granulomatous lesion (typically with accompanying leptomeningitis)

            clinical presentation—symptoms of intracranial mass lesion

            parenchymal lesion result of spread of leptomeningeal disease via Virchow-Robin spaces

- imaging appearance

    enhanced MR—preferred imaging modality for lesion detection (CT less sensitive for both meningeal and parenchymal involvement)

- differential diagnosis

    periventricular lesions

        multiple sclerosis (MS)

    diffuse leptomeningitis

        trauma

        tuberculosis

        bacterial meningitis

        meningeal carcinomatosis

1.23

Tuberculosis

- general information

    two main patterns of brain involvement

        parenchymal lesion (tuberculoma)

            up to 40% of all parenchymal mass lesions in brain are tuberculomas in developing countries

            most often solitary

serial imaging can demonstrate complete resolution following prolonged medical therapy

basal meningitis (more common than parenchymal involvement)

higher incidence in infants, children

can cause communicating hydrocephalus (due to blockage of CSF flow by inflammatory exudate)

can cause thrombosis, followed by infarction, of vessels coursing through basal cisterns—most commonly affected are small penetrating arteries to basal ganglia

- imaging appearance

granulomas—ring or nodular enhancement (capsule, often thicker than for pyogenic infection), center of lesion may be hypo- to hyperintense on T_2

MR > CT for detection, in particular for brainstem lesions

basal meningitis—abnormal contrast enhancement (MR > CT); high SI parenchymal abnormalities—ischemic or inflammatory change (often coexist on histologic exam)

1.251

Bacterial meningitis

- general information

meningitis = inflammation of meninges of brain or spinal cord

common organisms

general population—*Streptococcus pneumoniae, Neisseria meningitidis, Hemophilus influenzae*

neonate—*Escherichia coli,* other Gram-negative rods, group B streptococci

rapidly lethal without treatment

despite treatment, often complicated by infarction, deafness, intellectual impairment

- imaging appearance

uncomplicated cases—no detectable abnormalities

severe cases—bilateral subdural effusions (frontoparietal in location, slightly hyperintense to CSF on all pulse sequences, may contain linear foci of intermediate SI due to purulent material), abnormal leptomeningeal-contrast enhancement (MR > CT)

Viral meningitis

- imaging appearance (MR)

leptomeningeal or ependymal (ventricular lining) enhancement, due to inflammatory cell infiltration)

loss of cortical sulci, due to generalized brain swelling (cerebritis)

subdural fluid collections

1.2521

***Superficial siderosis** = hemosiderin deposition within macrophages in leptomeninges*

- general information

    cause—recurrent subarachnoid hemorrhage—usually from neoplasm (ependymoma, oligodendroglioma), aneurysm, vascular malformation, or (intraventricular) neonatal hemorrhage

    surface of cerebellum—most common site

    clinical presentation

    clinical syndrome only becomes manifest when deposition of hemosiderin is heavy (rare)

    sensorineural hearing loss, pyramidal tract signs, cerebellar dysfunction, progressive mental deterioration

    cranial nerve dysfunction—II, V, VII, VIII (severity of injury proportional to glial length of nerve)

    lesser degrees of hemosiderin deposition manifest little to no symptoms

- imaging appearance—high-field MR

    hypointensity of pial and arachnoid membranes on T_2

    well-demonstrated by GRE imaging (improved sensitivity to magnetic susceptibility)

1.253

Encephalitis

Herpes encephalitis (type 2)

- general information

    clinical presentation—microcephaly, vesiculopustular rash (infant exposed at birth due to vaginal delivery)

    causes widespread necrotizing meningoencephalitis

- imaging appearance

    CT

    early findings—patchy/widespread low attenuation (edema) in white matter; these areas increase rapidly in size and are accompanied by transient increased attenuation of cortical gray matter

    late findings—extensive white matter low attenuation (multicystic encephalomalacia), cortical atrophy, calcification (punctate/gyral)

    MR

    localized/generalized edema (early), evolving to multicystic encephalomalacia (late)

Herpes encephalitis (type 1)

- general information

    in older children and adults, herpes simplex virus type 1 (HSV-1) is most common cause of viral encephalitis nearly all adults have exposure to HSV-1 ("cold sores")

encephalitis is caused by reactivation of virus in trigeminal ganglion, with spread via cranial nerve V to meninges of anterior and middle cranial fossae—thus disease most commonly effects temporal and inferior frontal lobes

clinical presentation—headache, fever, seizures, confusion, behavioral changes

early diagnosis and treatment (acyclovir) critical to prevent hemorrhagic necrosis

- imaging appearance

  MR—much more sensitive than CT for detection of early disease

  T_2—edema (high SI) in cortex and white matter of involved area (temporal and/or frontal lobes, unilateral or bilateral)

  involvement commonly initially unilateral, with subsequent bilateral involvement not uncommon

---

1.254

Ependymitis

- general information

  definition—inflammation of ependymal lining of ventricle = ventriculitis

  etiology—complication of meningitis or encephalitis (bacterial), following surgery, with bacteremia, or contiguous extension of infection (otitis, sinusitis)

- imaging appearance

  MR—increased T_2 SI of periventricular white matter, ventricular lining, and CSF; enhancement of ventricular lining on T_1 following IV contrast

  differential diagnosis—intraventricular (ependymal) metastatic disease, which is usually more nodular

---

1.256

Brain abscess

- general information

  CT era brought marked improvement in survival, due to early diagnosis and better detection of treatment failures/complications

- imaging appearance—MR/CT

  characteristic features

  central necrosis (heterogeneous appearance)

  abscess capsule—low SI on T_2, enhances postcontrast on MR and CT—smooth, well defined, may be thinner medially (due to greater vascularity of gray matter vs. white matter)

  surrounding vasogenic edema

  gray-white matter junction location

  extraparenchymal spread—to CSF (ventricular/subarachnoid)

differential diagnosis—high-grade astrocytoma, large solitary necrotic metastasis

---

1.257

Epidural/subdural abscess

- imaging appearance

    MR—superior to CT for identification and definition of extent

    higher SI than CSF on both T_1 and T_2

    enhancement postcontrast

    IV contrast administration important for lesion detection

    displaced dura (epidural abscess only) seen as low SI interface on T_1 and T_2

    coronal scans may better display dural involvement (vs. axial), due to less partial volume imaging

---

1.2583

Sinus thrombosis

- general information

    etiology—infection, dehydration, trauma, neoplasia, hematologic abnormalities

    clinical presentation—headache, nausea, papilledema, lethargy (increased intracranial pressure)

    treatment—anticoagulants (with recanalization, long-term, of sinus)

- imaging appearance

    CT—hyperdense (precontrast), empty delta sign (postcontrast, due to enhancement of venous collateral channels which surround thrombosed sinus), hemorrhagic infarction

    MR

    acute (deoxyhemoglobin)—decreased intravascular SI (T_2)

    subacute (methemoglobin)—increased intravascular SI (T_1) (important to confirm same SI on two perpendicular planes, to avoid confusion with flow phenomena)

    postcontrast—enhancement of venous collaterals immediately surrounding sinus

    MRA—lack of flow on 2-D TOF or phase-contrast studies (both sensitive to slow flow)

Neoplasm, Neoplastic-like Condition ....

1.325

Esthesioneuroblastoma (olfactory neuroblastoma)

- general information

    arises from olfactory neuroepithelium which lines roof of nasal vault

    two-thirds of patients affected are between 10 and 40 years of age malignant, hematogenous metastases in more than 10%

treatment—surgical excision, with radiation therapy

- imaging appearance

    destructive-enhancing nasoethmoid soft tissue mass

    can extend into orbits, paranasal sinuses, or intracranially

    differential diagnosis—squamous cell carcinoma, metastasis, adenoid cystic carcinoma, osteogenic sarcoma, fibrous dysplasia, chronic infection

---

1.327

Chordoma

- general information

    slow-growing primary bone tumor, originating from remnant of primitive notochord (which can occur from clivus to sacrum)

    location—35% clivus, 50% sacrococcygeal, 15% vertebral body

    when intracranial, can extend to involve posterior and middle cranial fossae

    clinical presentation—men in third or fourth decades, with headache, facial pain, cranial nerve palsies, nasal stuffiness

    causes extensive bony destruction, locally aggressive (but histologically benign), rarely metastasize

    complete surgical resection rarely possible

- imaging appearance

    CT—calcification in 50%

    MR—well-defined, iso- to hypointense on T_1, high SI on T_2 (low SI septations common), enhance postcontrast

---

1.33

Calvarial metastasis

- imaging appearance

    MR—normal diploic space does not enhance (except for diploic veins), diploic metastases recognized by asymmetry of marrow space from side-to-side, with enhancement of lesion postcontrast, and destruction of outer or inner table with larger lesions

---

1.341

Leptomeningeal metastases

- general information

    detection relies principally on CSF cytology, which requires large volumes and multiple samples but is superior to both MR and CT

    poor prognosis

    neoplasms with propensity for leptomeningeal spread:

    1. primary brain—medulloblastoma, ependymoma, germinoma,

pineoblastoma, glioblastoma multiforme (GBM), oligodendroglioma, retinoblastoma

2. secondary—breast and lung carcinoma, melanoma, lymphoma, leukemia

common sites of involvement—quadrigeminal plate, perimesencephalic cistern, superior cerebellar cistern, ventricular ependyma, high-parietal subarachnoid space

- imaging appearance

  CT

  direct signs—abnormal contrast enhancement (nodular/smooth)

  indirect signs—hydrocephalus, obliteration of sylvian fissures/basal cisterns

  MR

  focal contrast enhancement of leptomeninges, may be edema within adjacent white/gray matter

  differential diagnosis—infection, trauma

1.343

Cerebral lymphoma

- general information

  <2% of all primary CNS tumors

  majority are primary in origin (however, in AIDS, equal number of primary and secondary lesions)

  increased incidence in immunodeficiency disorders (organ transplantation with immunosuppression, HIV infection)

  adults

  diagnosis by stereotactic biopsy

  treatment by radiation with steroids (median survival less than 24 months)

- imaging appearance

  CT/MR

  increased density (CT)

  large average lesion size (>2 cm), but smaller in AIDS

  common misconception—location in central white matter (only 30% in one series)

  prominent peritumoral edema

  homogeneous contrast enhancement (ring enhancement in immunosuppressed patients)

  multiple lesions (more common in AIDS) and/or subependymal spread seen in minority of cases

---

1.3611

Craniopharyngioma

- general information

  slow-growing benign tumor arising from remnants of Rathke's pouch

  clinical presentation

adults—headache, visual disturbances, hypopituitarism (due to compression of optic chiasm, hypothalamus or pituitary)

children—growth failure

age of incidence—two peaks—children (age 10), adults (age 35)

location

70% both intrasellar and suprasellar

20% solely suprasellar

most common suprasellar tumor

- imaging appearance

CT/MR

heterogeneous, with both cystic and solid components

cystic component higher SI than CSF on both T_1 and T_2 (protein, cholesterol, methemoglobin content)—in adult likely only slightly higher in SI on T_1 than brain, in children may be very high SI on T_1 (like fat)

solid components, and rim of cysts—display contrast enhancement, which assists in defining lesion extent

calcification on CT (80% of cases in children, 40% of cases in adults)

differential diagnosis—hypothalamic glioma, meningioma, metastatic disease, aneurysm, chordoma, sarcoidosis, Rathke's cleft cyst, teratoma, epidermoid, pituitary macroadenoma

---

1.3612

Colloid cyst

- general information

rare tumor of anterior third ventricle

thin fibrous capsule with epithelial lining

contents—secretory and breakdown products, including fat, blood, cholesterol, CSF

congenital origin, enlarge slowly—size ranges from mm to several cm, round

clinical presentation—usually not symptomatic until adult, cause hydrocephalus (obstruction of one or both foramina of Monro)

- imaging appearance—round lesion in anterosuperior third ventricle

CT—may be increased or decreased attenuation

MR—usually increased SI on T_1 (may be iso- or hypointense) and increased SI on T_2

1.3619

Arachnoid cyst

- general information

common (1% of all intracranial masses), benign, CSF-filled lesion

etiology—congenital (majority), inflammatory, trauma, subarachnoid hemorrhage location—middle cranial fossa (most common), brain convexity, retrocerebellar, perimesencephalic cistern

can be accompanying hypogenesis of temporal lobe, when located in middle cranial fossa

clinical presentation—most asymptomatic, can exhibit symptoms due to mass effect, seizures

- imaging appearance

CT—communicates with subarachnoid space, with filling by intrathecal contrast on delayed scans

MR—CSF SI on all pulse sequences

- differential diagnosis

epidermoid tumor—SI slightly different than CSF on MR, diffusion-weighted scans may also improve differentiation

cystic neoplasm—these demonstrate evidence of cyst wall, contrast enhancement, associated soft tissue mass, and/or surrounding edema

Leptomeningeal cyst

- rare complication of skull fracture in infant or child, usually parietal bone (can also occur following craniotomy)
- dural tear allows leptomeninges to herniate through fracture site, preventing normal bone healing
- subarachnoid fluid (and herniated brain) become trapped outside skull
- diagnosis often delayed (years following injury)

1.3621

Pineal region neoplasms

- general information

uncommon tumors, approximately 5% of childhood intracranial tumors, 1% of adult

four major groups

germ cell tumors (95% of tumors arising from pineal gland itself [can also arise in hypothalamus—suprasellar], occur in first three decades of life, male predominance, all prone to CSF seeding)

germinomas

most common pineal tumor

markedly radiosensitive

tumors of totipotential cells—endodermal sinus tumor (highly malignant), embryonal carcinoma (highly malignant), teratoma (if mature elements, good prognosis), choriocarcinoma

mixed lesions common

pineal parenchymal tumors (arise from neuroepithelial cells of pineal)

pineoblastoma—highly malignant, occurs in first two decades of life pineocytoma—benign, well-demarcated, noninvasive, slow-growing, presents in adults

glioma (with secondary invasion of pineal)

meningioma

clinical presentation—obstructive hydrocephalus (headache, vomiting, ataxia), paralysis of upward gaze (compression of tectum), endocrine abnormalities (with germ cell tumors)

- imaging appearance

    pineocytoma—(MR) heterogeneous, enhance following contrast; (CT) chunky calcifications

    germ cell tumors—(MR) contrast enhancement important to detect tumor seeding via CSF

- differential diagnosis

    pineal cyst—common normal variant (almost always asymptomatic), best visualized on sagittal images

        round, smoothly marginated, rarely >15 mm diameter, thin cyst wall

        homogeneous contents, usually CSF SI on all pulse sequences, can be slightly hyperintense to CSF on T_2 (best seen on scans with intermediate T_2-weighting)

        may demonstrate thin rim of enhancement

1.3622

Epidermoid

- general information

    benign congenital lesions, result from incomplete cleavage of neural from cutaneous ectoderm at time of neural tube closure, with retention of ectopic ectodermal cells in neural groove

    slow growth by desquamation of epithelial cells from lining (contain keratin, cholesterol)

    pliable, extends into and conforms to subarachnoid spaces—thus usually large when present clinically (adult), with surgical resection often incomplete

    location

        cerebellopontine angle (third most common lesion of CPA after acoustic neuroma and meningioma)

        middle cranial fossa

- imaging appearance

    CT—low density

    MR—SI slightly greater than CSF on both T_1 and T_2; imaging modality of choice for differentiation from arachnoid cyst (which has CSF SI on all pulse sequences); rarely high SI (fat SI) on T_1

Dermoid (intracranial)

- general information

    rare congenital lesion, occur in midline (vermis, pons, sella), differ from epidermoid by presence of skin appendages, hair follicles (dermal elements)

present in first three decades of life

"pearly" tumor—glistening white appearance of intact fibrous capsule at gross

clinical presentation—can rupture (with spread of fatty material into subarachnoid space and ventricular system), with meningeal signs, seizure, vasospasm; fat globules can be mobile

- imaging appearance

CT—hypodense (fat content)

MR—fat SI, with chemical shift artifact (differentiates high SI from methemoglobin)—usually very hyperintense on T_1, but this varies with fat content

Dermoid (intraorbital)

- general information

most common congenital orbital lesion, most common childhood orbital tumor

arise from sequestration of ectoderm along suture lines of orbital bones, usually frontozygomatic suture (superior temporal quadrant of orbit)

rupture not uncommon, with granulomatous reaction, calcification, scar

clinical presentation

first year of life—superficial, palpable, nontender nodule near lacrimal gland

children, adults—deep within orbit, with proptosis or displacement of globe

- imaging appearance

MR—well-circumscribed, spherical, heterogeneous SI (often with layering)—fat component dominates (high SI on T_1) and is pathognomonic for dermoid (vs. other lesions of orbit)

1.363

***Glial tumors ("glioma")**—graded histologically by degree of hypercellularity, pleomorphism, vascular proliferation, and presence of necrosis; on biopsy different portions of lesion commonly display different histology; further complication arises since lesions are not static histologically with time*

- MR recommended over CT for imaging, with superior depiction of tumor extent, cystic/necrotic change, and adjacent anatomy

Cerebellar astrocytoma

- general information

second most common posterior fossa tumor in childhood (primitive neuroectodermal tumor [PNET] = medulloblastoma slightly more common), 10–20% of all pediatric brain tumors, peak incidence in first decade of life low-grade, slow-growing, typically large at diagnosis

location—cerebellar hemisphere (80% cystic) or vermis (50% cystic)

cystic lesions—nodule (which enhances) is tumor, wall is non-neoplastic (must be differentiated from necrotic solid astrocytoma, in which wall will be neoplastic and enhancing)

clinical presentation—obstructive hydrocephalus (headache, nausea, ataxia)

- imaging appearance

  MR—SI of cystic component is slightly greater than CSF on all pulse sequences, due to protein content

- differential diagnosis

  hemangioblastoma

  arachnoid cyst (no enhancing component, CSF SI on all sequences)

  Dandy-Walker malformation

Astrocytoma

- general information

  three subtypes—as defined by National Brain Tumor Study Group (vs. classification by Kernohan's system into grades I–IV)

    low-grade

      peak incidence in third to fifth decades of life (earlier than glioblastoma multiforme [GBM]

      arise from glial cells in white matter

        common locations—reflect relative amount of white matter—frontal, temporal, parietal

        cortical involvement not uncommon

      clinical presentation—seizure, focal neurologic deficit, headache, nausea

      prognosis—better than GBM, better the younger the patient

    anaplastic astrocytoma (intermediate form between low-grade and glioblastoma multiforme)

    glioblastoma multiforme (GBM)—most common of the three lesions

      20% of all intracranial tumors

      hallmark on histologic exam—necrosis

      more advanced age of presentation, shorter duration of preoperative symptoms, shorter survival (vs. anaplastic astrocytoma)

      highly malignant, widely infiltrative (growth occurs along white matter tracts), with extension histologically of tumor beyond border marked on imaging by edema and abnormal contrast enhancement

      typically located in cerebral hemispheres, frontal most common followed by temporal

      multiple lobe involvement, ventricular rupture, spread via the corpus callosum to the opposite hemisphere ("butterfly" glioma) not uncommon clinical presentation—symptoms of increased intracranial pressure (headache, nausea/vomiting, changes in mentation, loss of consciousness), which result from CSF obstruction, edema, tissue destruction/irritation, and/or brain displacement

resistant to radiation/chemotherapy; gross total resection prolongs survival; median survival of 6 months

conversion of low-grade astrocytoma to anaplastic astrocytoma and subsequently to glioblastoma not uncommon, (incidence unknown, timing difficult to foretell in individual patient; however, in recurrences an increase in degree of malignancy is seen in majority)

- imaging appearance

low-grade astrocytoma

CT—calcifications in 25%, lesion may be isodense with brain (difficult to detect)

MR—well-defined, homogeneous, nonenhancing, little mass effect, minimal vasogenic edema

anaplastic astrocytomas

MR—less well defined, heterogeneous, may exhibit enhancement, moderate mass effect, vasogenic edema

IV contrast administration important for identification of recurrence or residual tumor (both with anaplastic astrocytomas and GBMs)—recurrent tumor usually enhances, even if preoperatively it did not

abnormal contrast enhancement does not differentiate between radiation necrosis (which usually occurs more than 1 year following treatment) and recurrent tumor

glioblastoma multiforme (GBM)

MR—poorly defined, greater heterogeneity (often gross central necrosis); thick, irregular enhancing ring, substantial mass effect, extensive white matter (vasogenic) edema, hemosiderin frequently noted (particularly on GRE scans)

differential diagnosis—metastatic disease, lymphoma, abscess

5% of patients with multiple tumor foci (either on first exam or on follow up)

multicentric—separate regions of tumor do not demonstrate micro- or macroscopic connection

multifocal—direct lesion continuity, or CSF spread, or local metastases

necrosis best defined on postcontrast scans

Oligodendroglioma

- general information

uncommon, 5% of intracranial gliomas

50% mixed (containing other glial elements)

young adults

peripheral location in cerebral hemispheres

most common—frontal lobe

arise in white matter, but can spread to cortex with obliteration of gray-white matter junction

can cause calvarial erosion—due to location and slow growth

infiltrating lesions (histologically)

treatment—surgical excision and radiation

- imaging appearance—well defined, without substantial edema

    CT

        calcification (nodular/linear) common

        half enhance (mildly) postcontrast

Ependymoma

- general information

    rare tumor, arising adjacent to ventricular system (most commonly fourth ventricle)—extra-axial in location

        when supratentorial, arise adjacent to lateral ventricles and often have cystic components

    slow-growing, benign

        commonly spread via CSF

    children, adolescents

    poor operative risk (location), thus poor prognosis

- imaging appearance

    MR

        solid, lobulated, heterogeneous (blood products, necrosis, vascularity)

Medulloblastoma

- general information

    primitive neuroectodermal tumor (PNET) of cerebellum

    most common posterior fossa neoplasm in childhood

        two-thirds of patients present in first decade (5–9 years)

        one-third present as young adults (20–24 years)

    arise from primitive neuroepithelial cells, majority in midline in roof of fourth ventricle

    tumor encroaches on or fills fourth ventricle

    highly malignant, with dissemination via CSF common (leptomeningeal metastases)

    clinical presentation—increased intracranial pressure (due to rapid tumor growth and obstructive hydrocephalus)

    radiosensitive, treatment by surgical resection and craniospinal radiation

- imaging appearance

    MR

        isointense with brain on T_1 and T_2

        half demonstrate intense homogeneous enhancement

        can demonstrate necrosis, cyst formation, calcification, or be eccentric in location (location in cerebellar hemispheres more common in older patient group)

- differential diagnosis (midline posterior fossa mass in child)

    astrocytoma

    ependymoma

Ganglion cell tumors

- general information

    spectrum from gangliocytoma (mature atypical neurons) to ganglioglioma (glial elements dominant)—incidence, macroscopic appearance, and biologic behavior similar; low grade

    temporal lobe most frequent location

    slow-growth, good demarcation

    clinical presentation

        longstanding symptoms

        <age 30

    treatment by surgical resection, relatively good prognosis

- imaging appearance

    MR/CT

        solid or predominantly cystic (often with mural nodule)

        little or no associated edema

        often contain calcifications (CT)

        half demonstrate contrast enhancement

Primitive neuroectodermal tumor (PNET)

- general information

    histology—undifferentiated cells resembling germinal matrix

    highly malignant—propensity to invade locally, disseminate via CSF, and metastasize outside CNS

    second most common brain tumor in pediatrics (supra- and infratentorial together) following astrocytoma

    clinical presentation—childhood; headache, nausea, increasing head circumference, papilledema, seizures, neurologic deficit

- imaging appearance

    CT/MR

        large well-circumscribed mass

        frontal or parietal location

        dominant cystic component, with enhancing soft tissue along periphery—hemorrhage within cyst not uncommon (can be reason for clinical presentation)

        calcification (CT) and necrosis—common

Choroid plexus papilloma

- general information

    rare, malignant transformation unusual, leptomeningeal seeding can occur both communicating and noncommunicating hydrocephalus can occur, the first due to excessive production of CSF, the latter due to outlet obstruction

location

lateral ventricle—children

fourth ventricle—adults

cauliflowerlike mass (on gross)

treatment by surgical resection

- imaging appearance

CT/MR

highly vascular, with signal voids due to blood flow (MR)

intense homogeneous enhancement

- differential diagnosis—lateral ventricle neoplasm

meningioma

subependymoma

giant cell astrocytoma

lymphoma

metastasis

Brainstem (pontine) glioma

- general information

histology—pilocystic astrocytoma, tendency to undergo anaplastic change

location—predominantly pons, although contiguous involvement of brainstem common

exophytic extension and CSF seeding common

clinical presentation—childhood, adolescence

treatment—radiation (palliative)

Optic nerve glioma

- general information

histology—low-grade, well-differentiated astrocytes

most common cause of optic nerve enlargement

can extend posteriorly to involve chiasm and optic tracts, then nonresectable

clinical presentation

75% in first decade (peak at age 5)

visual disturbances, proptosis

association with neurofibromatosis type 1 (then often bilateral)

clinical course—relatively benign

- imaging appearance

CT/MR

fusiform enlargement of optic nerve

slight hyperintensity on T_2 (MR)

- differential diagnosis (optic nerve enlargement)

  meningioma

  inflammation (optic neuritis)

  leukemia, lymphoma

Tectal glioma

- general information

  can cause obstruction of cerebral aqueduct, anywhere along its length

- imaging appearance

  MR

  bulbous mass of tectum (= colliculi)

  high SI on T_2 (vs. benign aqueductal stenosis, which can manifest thickening, but not a bulbous mass, with a thin rim of periaqueductal hyperintensity)

  sagittal-thin section imaging important for depiction of aqueduct

- differential diagnosis (aqueductal narrowing)

  congenital

  stenosis

  septum

  gliosis, inflammation

  mass lesion

1.364

Nerve, nerve sheath tumors—schwannomas account for 8% of all primary intracranial tumors, with 90% from cranial nerve VIII (acoustic) and the next most common nerve involved being cranial nerve V (trigeminal). Lesions of other nerves (vagus, glossopharyngeal) and multiplicity of involvement suggest neurofibromatosis

Acoustic (VIII) neuroma (schwannoma)

- general information

  histology—benign tumor of Schwann cells

  arise from vestibular division of eighth cranial nerve

  displaces rather than incorporates the nerve (like all schwannomas)

  location

  most common extra-axial tumor of cerebellopontine angle (80%)

  majority have intra- and extracanalicular component, centered on porus acusticus

  up to 35% purely intracanalicular

  clinical presentation

  35–60 years of age

unilateral sensorineural hearing loss, tinnitus

large tumors may compress brainstem, with ataxia, vertigo

- imaging appearance

    MR (modality of choice)

    extracanalicular portion is usually round (vs. plaque-like appearance of meningioma)

    enlargement of porus acusticus

    hypo- to isointense on T_1 with brain, iso- to hyperintense on T_2

    calcification, cysts, hemorrhage, necrosis can cause heterogeneous appearance

    intense enhancement following IV contrast administration—important for identification of small intracanalicular lesions

    important to differentiate from enhancement of seventh or eighth cranial nerve from inflammation alone (for example with Bell's palsy)

- differential diagnosis

    meningioma (enlargement of porus acusticus, and extension into IAC are rare with meningiomas)

    presence of enhancing dural "tail" (MR) not specific for meningioma vs. acoustic neuroma

    epidermoid

    other less common lesions—fifth or seventh nerve schwannoma, glomus jugulare, arachnoid cyst, exophytic brainstem glioma

Trigeminal (V) schwannoma

- general information

    location

    arise from gasserian ganglion, most confined to middle cranial fossa

    minority extend into both middle and posterior fossae, with dumbbell shape (constriction where nerve penetrates dura at petrous apex)

    can erode petrous bone when large

    clinical presentation—fifth nerve is chief sensory nerve to face and motor nerve for mastication

    facial pain

    atrophy of the muscles of mastication (masseter, temporalis, medial and lateral pterygoids)

- imaging appearance

    MR superior to CT due to soft tissue detail and lack of bone artifact

- differential diagnosis (lesions involving cavernous sinus with perineural extent)

    head and neck tumors (squamous cell, adenoid cystic carcinoma)

    lymphoma

    meningioma

1.3651

Hemangioblastoma

- general information

  histology—rare tumor of embryonic vascular elements

  usually solitary, located in cerebellum (less commonly in cervical spinal cord)

  most common primary cerebellar tumor in adult

  etiology—sporadic (80%) or as part of von Hippel-Lindau syndrome (latter patients typically have multiple lesions and present as children)

  clinical presentation—headache, papilledema, ataxia

- imaging appearance

  CT/MR

  sharply marginated cystic mass with peripheral-enhancing mural nodule (which abuts pia mater)

  SI of cyst is slightly greater than CSF on both T_1 and T_2 (due to protein content)

  cyst wall is non-neoplastic

  enlarged associated blood vessels often noted

  one-third of lesions are solid (also sharply marginated, enhancing, with abnormal vascularity)—usually <1 cm diameter

- differential diagnosis (cystic cerebellar mass in adult)

  metastasis

  abscess

  astrocytoma

1.366

Meningioma

- clinical presentation

  common "incidental" finding (<1 cm lesion diameter)

  when symptomatic—due to mass effect on vital structures

- pathogenesis

  most common benign intracranial tumor (15% of all intracranial tumors in adults)

  most common extra-axial adult tumor

  multiple in 6–8% of cases

  peak age incidence—fifth decade

  rare under age of 30

  occurrence rate 1:2 (male:female)

  slow-growing

  histopathologic subtypes

  fibroblastic

  transitional

syncytial

angioblastic

- common locations

parasagittal (falx)

convexity

sphenoid wing

parasellar, suprasellar

> differential diagnosis in suprasellar region includes—pituitary macroadenoma, craniopharyngioma, optic nerve glioma, aneurysm, metastasis, chordoma, hypothalamic glioma, infundibular tumor

olfactory groove

tentorium cerebelli

petrous ridge

cerebellopontine angle

> most common extra-axial tumor in this location is an acoustic neuroma

foramen magnum

intraventricular (rare—1%)

> location—atrium of lateral ventricles, or at foramen of Monro

> most common tumor of atrium of lateral ventricle (there supplied by anterior choroidal artery)

> increased incidence in neurofibromatosis

> frequently calcified (calcification not a distinguishing point, as this is also seen in ependymomas and choroid plexus papillomas)

- imaging appearance

general

> broad based along bony or dural surface

> cause displacement of adjacent brain tissue

> benign, but can invade venous sinuses and bone

plain film

> bony hyperostosis (especially en plaque type)

CT

> 25% calcified

> 75% hyperdense

MR

> homogeneous SI typical—inhomogeneity when present due to calcification, vascularity, necrosis, or cystic changes

> iso- or hyperintense to brain on T_2, iso- or hypointense on T_1—commonly isointense with brain on both T_1- and T_2-weighted images

> some tumors have no surrounding edema, others elicit extensive edema

> intense homogeneous contrast enhancement (important for detection of small lesions)

dural "tail" (linear-enhancing thickening of meninges extending away from tumor) common (60%)—but not specific for meningioma

multiplanar imaging useful to confirm extra-axial location

arteriography

prolonged vascular stain

En plaque meningioma

- general information

  grow along planes of leptomeninges (not globular)

  common locations—sphenoid ridge, cortical convexity

- imaging features

  difficult to detect on CT (due to bony artifact) and on unenhanced MR

  marked hyperostosis of adjacent bone not uncommon, often disproportionate with tumor size

- differential diagnosis

  dural-based metastases

Perioptic (optic nerve) meningioma

- clinical presentation

  visual loss, proptosis

- pathogenesis

  arise from optic sheath

  one-third of tumors of optic nerve, sheath

  5% of primary orbital tumors

  third to fifth decades

  80% in women

- imaging appearance

  CT >> MR for detection of calcification

  MR—mild enhancement of intraorbital tumor, intense enhancement of intracranial tumor

  perineural enhancement ("tram-track")—classically described, not pathognomonic

- differential diagnosis—optic nerve glioma (90% < age 20), leukemia, lymphoma, metastases, pseudotumor, neurofibroma

Hemangiopericytoma

- pathogenesis

  arise from embryonic vascular elements (angioblasts)—as do angioblastic meningiomas and hemangioblastomas

  5% of all tumors which involve the meninges

  high cellularity, extremely vascular, malignant

  high recurrence rate

  systemic metastases in 20%

  peak incidence—fourth to sixth decades

- imaging appearance

  due to location, tendency to compress adjacent brain—often mistaken for meningioma

---

1.367

Hemorrhage, hematoma

- general information

  pathogenesis

  vascular malformations—common cause of spontaneous hemorrhage in normotensive young adults

(MR description below is for high-field scanners—1.5 T; at lower fields, susceptibility effects which cause a decrease in SI are not generally evident)

Hyperacute hematoma (oxyhemoglobin)—0 to 12 hours in age

- imaging appearance

  CT

  hyperdense

  MR (note—imaging appearance is nonspecific)

  T_2—high SI

  T_1—isointense (or slightly hypointense) to brain

Acute hematoma (deoxyhemoglobin)

- imaging appearance

  MR

  T_2—low SI—this appearance develops sooner and is more pronounced at high (1.5 T) vs. mid- or low-field strengths

  T_1—isointense to brain

Subacute hematoma (methemoglobin)

- imaging appearance

  MR

  T_2—low SI when intracellular (early subacute, intracellular methemoglobin), high SI when extracellular (late subacute, extracellular methemoglobin)

  T_1—high SI

Chronic hematoma (hemosiderin and ferritin)

- histochemical studies

  both hemosiderin and ferritin are present in chronic brain hemorrhage

- imaging appearance

  ultimate appearance dependent on whether central fluid collection is resorbed or not

  if resorbed, only a hemosiderin and ferritin cleft will be left

  if not resorbed, will be central fluid collection with high SI on both T_1 and T_2, surrounded by hemosiderin and ferritin rim

MR (appearance of cleft or rim)

T_2—low SI

T_1—isointense to slightly hypointense to brain

- comments (hematomas)

often hematomas do not follow the above characteristic patterns on MR—additional factors such as dilution and clotting can be important

edema (high SI on T_2) is present, surrounding the hematoma, in hyperacute, acute and early subacute stages

Subarachnoid hemorrhage

- CT

modality of choice in evaluation for acute subarachnoid hemorrhage (high attenuation)

can be negative in patients with subarachnoid hemorrhage, due to either time delay between hemorrhage and imaging or small quantity of blood

- MR

equivalent to CT for detection of subarachnoid blood less than 24 hours of age—T_1 shortening produces accentuated hyperintensity of CSF on T_2-weighted scans—but observation of this finding requires attention to film and windowing

superior to CT for detection of subacute subarachnoid hemorrhage—with high SI seen on T_1 scans (clot, methemoglobin)

- arteriography

very small percent of patients with ruptured brain aneurysm will have normal angiogram, despite presence of subarachnoid blood, due to vasospasm (causing nonfilling)

Intraventricular hemorrhage

- general information

in newborns, often result of subependymal germinal matrix bleed, with rupture of ependyma

germinal matrix—highly vascular, fragile growth zone in subependyma; decreases in size with increasing fetal age (involutes by 34 weeks of gestation)

majority of infants with germinal matrix bleed are premature (<32 weeks)

grades of germinal matrix hemorrhage (higher grade, worse prognosis)

grade I—confined to subependyma

grade II—extends into nondilated ventricle

grade III—intraventricular hemorrhage with ventricular dilatation

grade IV—with associated parenchymal hemorrhage

- imaging appearance

MR

SI on T_1 and T_2 dependent on age of hemorrhage

MRA—on MIP from TOF MRA, clot (methemoglobin) within ventricles may be visualized as high SI and potentially misinterpreted as blood flow

1.369

Lipoma

- clinical presentation—most asymptomatic
- etiology—rare congenital malformation (persistence/maldifferentiation of meninx primitiva—a mesenchymal derivative of neural crest)
- characteristic locations (within brain)

  interhemispheric (most common, 45%), quadrigeminal plate or superior cerebellar (25%), suprasellar or interpeduncular (14%), cerebellopontine angle (9%) and sylvian (5%) cisterns
- 55% associated with brain malformations

  corpus callosal lipomas—50% associated with agenesis
- imaging appearance

  intracranial vessels and nerves course through the lipoma (not displaced)

  MR—hyperintense on T_1, lower SI on T_2 (characteristic of fat), chemical shift artifact seen in frequency-encoding direction (at interface with brain or CSF)

  differential diagnosis—falx ossification

1.37

Pituitary microadenoma

- pathology

  prolactinomas

  most common secretory lesion of pituitary, 90% women

  clinical symptoms—irregular menses, amenorrhea, galactorrhea

  serum prolactin level >300 µg/L diagnostic, level >100 µg/L indeterminate

  treatment—dopamine-agonist drugs (bromocriptine)
- imaging appearance

  CT

  asymmetry of pituitary gland (focal convexity), sellar floor abnormality, infundibular displacement (all also well visualized by MR)

  MR twice as sensitive as CT for lesion detection

  MR

  normal pituitary—following IV contrast, there is immediate, prominent enhancement of infundibulum, anterior pituitary, cavernous sinus (maximum approximately 1–2 min postinjection)

  pituitary adenomas (macro- and micro-)—later peak of enhancement with slower washout—utility of early postcontrast scans for lesion identification—greater relative enhancement of normal pituitary vs. adenoma

thin section (≤3 mm, coronal and sagittal images), small FOV, high-field (1.5 T, high SNR), and T_1-weighting—important for lesion identification

delayed postcontrast scans of no additional benefit

differential diagnosis (small intrasellar lesion)—Rathke's cleft cyst

Pituitary macroadenoma (>10 mm diameter)

- pathology

  frequently nonsecretory

  clinical symptoms—caused by pressure on adjacent structures—visual loss (optic chiasm splayed, compressed—most common visual field defect is bitemporal hemianopsia), hypopituitarism

  treatment

  bromocriptine (for lesions which secrete prolactin)—causes shrinkage

  transsphenoidal resection

- imaging appearance

  MR (technique of choice, vs. CT)

  isointense with brain on T_1 and T_2, uniform moderate-contrast enhancement (also improved delineation of mass, in particular from cavernous sinus)

  suprasellar extension—preceded by sella expansion; tumor often dumbbell in shape (constricted by diaphragma sellae/circle of Willis)

  cavernous sinus invasion (not uncommon)—carotid artery encasement only reliable sign

  differential diagnosis—intrasellar meningioma, pituitary metastasis

Pituitary apoplexy

- sudden infarction (bland or hemorrhagic) within normal gland or tumor

  sudden enlargement of gland/compression of adjacent structures—produces symptoms

1.371

Ocular melanoma

- clinical presentation—decreased visual acuity, pain
- nonimaging features

  uveal tract (choroid, ciliary body, iris) melanoma—most common primary intraocular neoplasm in adults

  peak age incidence—50 years

  uncommon in children

  unilateral lesion, retinal detachment common

- imaging

    usually initially diagnosed via ophthalmoscopy (true of all ocular tumors)

        ophthalmoscopy—cannot distinguish melanoma from other tumors or retinal detachment

    MR—role—characterization, definition of extent

        characteristic SI of melanotic melanomas (due to stable free radicals within melanin)—markedly hyperintense on T_1, markedly hypointense on T_2 relative to vitreous

            differential diagnosis—same SI seen with choroidal nevus and retinoblastoma (nearly always in children, with 100% containing calcification by CT)

        can differentiate from subretinal fluid (retinal detachment)—very high SI on T_2

1.38

Brain metastases

- nonimaging features

    surgical resection combined with radiotherapy for single brain metastases prolongs survival, improves quality of life

    lung cancer, specifically adenocarcinoma and large cell—early preferential metastasis to CNS

    treatment options—surgical resection (single lesion), stereotactic radiation (for two to six lesions), whole brain radiation

- imaging appearance

    location at gray-white matter junction, large amount of associated cerebral edema—common features

    MR (with IV contrast is superior to double-dose delayed CT for lesion detection)

        IV contrast enhancement (mandatory)—increases lesion detection (particularly for small tumor nodules—not all lesions manifest a T_2 abnormality or surrounding edema), and improves depiction of necrosis

            detectability further improved by high-contrast dose (0.3 mmol/kg vs. 0.1 mmol/kg)

                identification of all lesions important for choice of therapy with recent advent of stereotactic radiation therapy (gamma-knife)

Metastatic melanoma

- imaging appearance—influenced by melanin and hemorrhage, either of which may be present

    MR—nonhemorrhagic melanotic melanoma—marked hyperintensity on T_1 (due to paramagnetic effect of melanin)

        differential diagnosis—other hemorrhagic metastases—renal cell carcinoma, bronchogenic carcinoma, thyroid carcinoma, choriocarcinoma

Meningeal carcinomatosis

- imaging appearance

    MR (with contrast enhancement) > CT for lesion detection

    imaging may be negative despite positive cytology (CSF)

Effect of Trauma ....

1.432

Epidural hematoma

- general information

    dura = periosteum of inner table—strongly adherent to skull

    epidural hematoma accumulates between inner table of skull and dura (typically due to skull fracture with laceration of blood vessel)

    most common—middle meningeal artery laceration (temporal/parietal bone fracture)

    less common (posterior fossa)—transverse sinus laceration (occipital bone fracture)

    clinical presentation—may not become symptomatic for several hours (lucid interval), often with acute rapidly progressive deterioration

- imaging appearance

    biconvex, elliptical fluid collection, which can cross the midline (falx) and the tentorium

    venous sinuses displaced away from skull

    CT—exam of choice (quick, relatively insensitive to motion, no difficulty with life-support systems)

    MR—more sensitive for coexisting parenchymal brain injuries, as well as for subacute hemorrhage

1.433

Subdural hematoma

- general information

    dura lacks a blood-brain barrier, thus macrophages may freely enter (removing blood products)

- imaging appearance

    convex inward border

    MR

    can identify age of lesion, due to SI appearance (deoxyhemoglobin vs. intracellular methemoglobin vs. extracellular methemoglobin)

    chronic subdurals differ in appearance from parenchymal hematomas—isointense (to slightly hypointense) with brain on T_1 and do not demonstrate hemosiderin deposition (unless recurrent)

1.435

Trauma

- general information
    - cortical contusion = bruise of brain's surface
        - inferior frontal and temporal poles of brain—particularly vulnerable
        - coup—injury lies beneath area of impact
        - contrecoup—occurs remote from injury, in direct line opposite site of impact, caused by acceleration effects
        - four types of intra-axial traumatic brain lesions, based on location
            - diffuse axonal injury—most common
                - due to shear-strain forces
                - multiple, small ovoid foci in white matter, typically at gray-white matter junction, 20% with hemorrhagic component
                - most common location—parasagittal white matter of frontal lobe and white matter of temporal lobes
                - second most common location—corpus callosum, specifically splenium (usually with lobar involvement)
                - intraventricular hemorrhage—common
            - cortical contusion
            - subcortical gray matter injury
            - primary brainstem injury
- imaging appearance
    - MR = CT for detection of hemorrhagic parenchymal injury
        - old lesions contain hemosiderin, with low SI on T_2 (MR)
    - MR > CT for detection of nonhemorrhagic lesions and extra-axial fluid collections
        - acute lesions—low SI on T_1, high SI on T_2 (edema)
        - chronic lesions—high SI on T_2 (gliosis, demyelination)
    - angiography
        - blunt trauma—can result in intimal tear, pseudoaneurysm, dissection, thrombosis, or embolization
        - penetrating trauma—can result in intimal tear, laceration, pseudoaneurysm, arteriovenous fistula, or occlusion

1.4371

Chronic head injury

- imaging appearance
    - findings include shear injury, encephalomalacia (cystic changes—end result of cortical contusion), generalized atrophy, damage at gray-white matter junction, old hemorrhage

1.47

Radiation white matter changes

- general information
    - early changes—white matter vasogenic edema (damage to capillary endothelium)—limited clinical consequence
    - late changes—axonal demyelination with increased water content
        - more common in elderly patients, and with higher total radiation dose
        - time of onset from treatment varies, after single dose—seen by 7 months
- imaging appearance (late changes)
    - MR—diffuse, symmetric white matter hyperintensity on T_2, affects majority of periventricular white matter (spares corpus callosum)

Radiation necrosis

- general information
    - increased incidence with increased radiation dose
- imaging appearance
    - MR—region of T_2 hyperintensity, with contrast enhancement
    - cannot be distinguished by imaging alone (CT or MR) from recurrent tumor

1.494

Dural arteriovenous fistula

- general information
    - acquired vascular malformation, most common in posterior fossa, usually involve venous sinus
    - etiology—occlusion of venous sinus, with attempt at recanalization along wall of sinus leading to numerous direct connections between small feeding arteries and venous drainage
    - clinical complications—venous infarction, parenchymal hemorrhage, subdural hematoma
    - carotid artery-cavernous sinus fistula (subset of dural arteriovenous fistula)
        - traumatic laceration of ICA, or rupture of aneurysm, within cavernous sinus
        - clinical presentation—pulsatile exophthalmos, bruit, diplopia
- imaging appearance
    - MR/CT—large superficial dural-based veins, without parenchymal nidus
        - carotid artery-cavernous sinus fistula—enlargement of cavernous sinus and superior ophthalmic vein (due to increased flow, or thrombosis)
    - angiography—often visualizes the small feeding arteries (these are not see n by MR)

Metabolic, Endocrine, Toxic.............................

1.512

Acromegaly

- general information

    caused by excess of growth hormone in adults, usually due to pituitary adenoma, resulting in bony and soft tissue overgrowth

    surgical excision is treatment of choice—recurrent tumor (and symptoms) not uncommon

- imaging appearance

    paranasal sinus enlargement, prognathism (forward projection of jaw), skull thickening (enlarged diploic space)

1.5911

Anoxic brain injury

- general information

    etiology—inadequate oxygen to brain, either due to hypoxia (decreased blood oxygen content) or ischemia (hypoperfusion)

- imaging appearance

    brain not affected uniformly

    gray matter (neurons) more vulnerable than white matter, with watershed zones between arterial circulations particularly vulnerable

    highly susceptible (anoxia)—hippocampus, cerebral cortex, cerebellum, caudate, putamen

    less susceptible (anoxia)—globus pallidus, thalamus, hemispheric white matter, brainstem

Total parenteral nutrition (TPN)

- imaging appearance

    MR—long-term TPN may give high SI in globus pallidus on T_1, due to deposition of paramagnetic trace elements, in particular manganese

Other Generalized Systemic Disorders................

1.61

Systemic lupus erythematosus (SLE)

- general information

    40% of SLE patients clinically demonstrate CNS involvement—seizures, stroke

- imaging appearance

    MR > CT for lesion detection

lesions can be noted in gray matter (alone), white matter (subcortical or deep) alone, or in both gray and white matter (territorial infarct)

differential diagnosis—MS, neurosarcoidosis, other vasculitides

resolution of some lesions (excluding the territorial infarcts) has been noted on follow-up MR

1.62194

Moyamoya

- general information

    etiology—occlusion or stenosis of terminal ICA, together with proximal anterior and middle cerebral artery branches

    most common in children

    increased incidence in Japanese

- imaging appearance

    hemispheric and subcortical (centrum semiovale) infarctions

    bilateral, multiple, predominantly in carotid circulation in watershed regions

    infarcts also described in caudate, putamen, globus pallidus, internal capsule

    network of small anastomotic vessels at base of brain—"cloud of smoke"

1.663

Langerhans' cell (eosinophilic) granulomatosis

- general information—disease of childhood

    unifocal form—predominantly males, solitary osteolytic lesion, treatment by excision

    multifocal form—multiple bony lesions, diabetes insipidus in one-third due to hypothalamic involvement, benign (but treated with chemotherapy)

- imaging appearance

    diploic space lesions (skull) well visualized by CT and MR

    resolution of hypothalamic lesions has been observed with effective therapy

Vascular Disorders...

1.729

Vertebrobasilar dolichoectasia

- general information

    definition

        elongation ("dolicho")—presence of basilar artery lateral to clivus or dorsum sellae, or bifurcating above suprasellar cistern

        distention ("ectasia")—basilar artery diameter >4.5 mm

clinical presentation

isolated nerve involvement (third, sixth, or seventh)

more likely with tortuous, but normal caliber basilar artery

multiple neurologic deficits—combination of cranial nerve deficits (due to compression) and CNS deficits (due to compression or ischemia)

more likely with ectatic basilar artery

- imaging appearance

arteriography—if required, digital subtraction techniques advised due to risk of brainstem ischemia

MR—asymptomatic deformity of pons, due to basilar artery ectasia, common incidental finding in elderly population

---

1.733

Mycotic aneurysm

- general information

caused by septic emboli

located peripherally (vs. congenital aneurysms)

"mycotic"—term used traditionally to refer to both bacterial and fungal aneurysms, with majority bacterial

treatment—medical (antibiotics) vs. surgery, former favored

serial angiography recommended—looking for enlargement

high mortality rate with rupture

- imaging appearance

CT/MR—enhancing mass with surrounding cerebral edema (nonspecific)

MRA may depict flow within lesion

1.736

Aneurysm (berry, saccular)

- general information

1–8% of population have intracranial berry aneurysms

incidence higher in patients with a relative having a ruptured aneurysm

multiple in 15–20% of cases, increasing age correlates with increased number

associated with adult polycystic kidney disease, Marfan's syndrome, aortic coarctation

clinical presentation—subarachnoid hemorrhage

intracranial location—arterial branching sites

posterior communicating artery (PCA)—20–30%

anterior communicating artery (ACA)—30%

middle cerebral artery (MCA) bifurcation—20%

posterior fossa circulation—15%

most common at apex (dome) of basilar artery—can compress cranial nerves (but usually present with subarachnoid hemorrhage)

next most common—origin of posterior inferior cerebellar artery (PICA)

- imaging appearance

MR—diagnosis more definitive, due to observation of flow effects and use of MRA, than with CT

spin-echo technique

size, residual lumen, location well depicted

arterial flow causes pulsation artifacts, which serve to confirm vascular nature of lesion

MRA

technique—3-D TOF

exception—giant intracranial aneurysms may be better depicted with 2-D TOF, due to slow flow

permits detection of aneurysms in circle of Willis as small as 3 mm

inferior spatial resolution compared to conventional contrast arteriography

---

1.7362

Giant intracranial aneurysm

- general information

definition—saccular aneurysm with diameter >25 mm

2.5–5% of all intracranial aneurysms

clinical presentation—space-occupying lesion, with visual changes, cranial nerve palsies, and/or seizures (but rupture can occur)

location—most common from cavernous or supraclinoid ICA, or at bifurcation of MCA

parasellar location—differential diagnosis—meningioma, craniopharyngioma, pituitary adenoma

treatment is surgical, with approaches including ligation of neck of aneurysm, use of intravascular balloons, and ICA ligation

- imaging appearance

MR—complex, due to presence of both flowing blood and thrombus (which may be layered); presence of pulsation artifacts may offer clue to nature of lesion

2-D or phase-contrast MRA best for detection of full extent of aneurysm (slow flow in lumen)

1.74

Internal carotid artery (ICA) dissection

- general information

clinical presentation (nonspecific)—neck/face pain, Horner's syndrome (ptosis, miosis, anhidrosis) treatment—surgery not indicated unless pseudoaneurysm is present, or deficits are progressive; anticoagulation is important to prevent strokes from embolus arising at site of dissection

if complete occlusion does not occur, most spontaneously resolve (within months)

- imaging appearance

    MR—quite sensitive for detection of subacute dissection

    crescent of abnormal SI (subacute hematoma)—hyperintense on T_1, hyper- or hypointense on T_2 (extra- vs. intracellular methemoglobin)

    compromise of vessel lumen well-depicted

    absence of normal flow void on spin-echo images within carotid siphon can be due to either slow flow or occlusion

---

1.75

Arteriovenous malformation (AVM)

- general information

    clinical presentation—seizure (common), neurologic deficits, headache, hemorrhage (parenchymal or subarachnoid)

    risk of hemorrhage is 2–3% per year, with each episode having 30% risk of death

    most common symptomatic vascular malformation of brain (other types—venous and cavernous angiomas, capillary telangiectasia)

    nidus is tangle of tightly packed dilated, tortuous arteries and veins, without an intervening capillary network—result is arteriovenous shunting

    aneurysms of feeding arteries in 7–9%

    congenital, present between 20 and 40 years of age, 80% symptomatic by age 50

    location

    90% supratentorial—most common within frontal and parietal lobes

    most involve peripheral branches of ACA or MCA

- imaging appearance

    CT—mass lesion, with little mass effect or surrounding edema, calcification in 25–50%

    MR—AVMs well depicted on conventional spin echo MR (due to flow phenomena), with TOF MRA used to demonstrate nidus, enlarged arterial feeding vessels, and enlarged draining veins (on occasion, a small AVM will be visualized only on MRA, not on spin echo)

    spin echo—multiple serpiginous structures, most with low SI due to rapid flow

    size of nidus, precise anatomic location of lesion best evaluated by MR

    angiography—remains the standard for detection and delineation of AVMs (important for evaluation of arterial feeders and venous drainage)

Venous angioma

- general information

  developmental anomaly of venous drainage of periependymal zones—a collection of abnormal veins

  peripheral dilated medullary veins (stellate or umbrella configuration = caput medusae), usually draining toward ventricular wall (in supratentorial lesions), converging to a central dilated draining vein, which runs in a transhemispheric course

  most common asymptomatic vascular malformation of brain

  symptoms, when they do occur, include headache, seizure, vertigo

  hemorrhage and venous infarction are rare complications, seen more with posterior fossa lesions

  location—frontal lobe 40%, cerebellum 25%; usually solitary

- imaging appearance

  MR—with contrast enhancement (and MRA) has replaced CT and conventional angiography for diagnosis

  intense enhancement following IV-contrast administration (important for detection)

Cavernous angioma

- general information

  clinical presentation—seizures, hemorrhage, or space-occupying mass

  present in third to fifth decades, 75% supratentorial (often subcortical), multiplicity common (25%)

  prone to spontaneous hemorrhage, treatment by surgical resection

  histology—honeycomb of vascular spaces, separated by fibrous strands, without intervening normal parenchyma

- imaging appearance

  CT—high density, calcification

  MR—mixed low and high SI on both T_1 and T_2, with hemosiderin (hypointense on T_2) rim; contrast enhancement common

  imaging with techniques sensitive to magnetic susceptibility (T_2^*), such as GRE, important for improved lesion detection

  angiography—occult or "cryptic"

1.781

Infarction

- general information

  in young, often embolic in etiology (valve vegetations, left atrial thrombus due to atrial fibrillation)

  in elderly, typically due to atherosclerosis, which most commonly effects carotid bifurcation, ICA, and MCA

  known complication of drug ingestion or abuse

anticoagulants, oral contraceptives, ergot alkaloids, cocaine, amphetamines

cocaine and amphetamines—cause vasoconstriction, vasculitis

clinical presentation—acute neurologic deficit

anatomical location

precentral gyrus (primary motor strip)—hemiparesis

anterior to primary motor cortex and above Sylvian fissure (Broca's area)—expressive aphasia

posterior superior temporal lobe (Wernicke's area)—infarction in dominant hemisphere causes receptive aphasia (loss of intellectual functions associated with language or symbolism)

arterial territories—cerebral (infarctions, other than lacunae, involve gray and white matter in a discrete vascular territory)

MCA—most common

PCA—next most common, following MCA

posterior cerebral artery can originate from tip of basilar artery, or from internal carotid artery (fetal origin)

supplies posterior-inferior temporal lobe, occipital lobe, medial parietal lobe, and portions of the brainstem, thalamus, and internal capsule

ACA—rare (3% of cerebral infarctions)

anterior cerebral artery supplies anterior putamen, caudate nucleus, hypothalamus, corpus callosum, medial surface of hemisphere

lacunar infarction

small, deep cerebral infarcts, most frequently seen with hypertension

result from occlusion of small penetrating arteries arising from the major cerebral arteries

most commonly involve basal ganglia, internal capsule, thalamus, and brainstem

arterial territories—posterior fossa and brainstem

pons

supplied by penetrating arteries (thalamoperforators) from basilar tip and proximal PCA

infarcts of pons are most frequently unilateral, paramedian and sharply marginated at midline

bilateral infarction does occur (still paramedian)

lateral pontine infarcts uncommon

differential diagnosis for bilateral pontine infarct on imaging—MS, central pontine myelinolysis, pontine glioma

medulla

lateral medullary infarction = Wallenberg's syndrome

clinical presentation—dysarthria, dysphagia, vertigo, nystagmus, ipsilateral Horner's syndrome, contralateral loss of pain and temperature sense (over the body)

acute phase—respiratory and cardiovascular complications are major hazards

has been reported following chiropractic neck manipulation (due to dissection of vertebral artery near atlantoaxial joint)

arteries supplying lateral medulla usually arise from distal vertebral artery, but can originate from PICA (thus, lateral medullary syndrome sometimes seen in patients with PICA infarction)

medial medullary infarction

clinical presentation—contralateral hemiparesis (sparing the face)

posterior inferior cerebellar artery (PICA)

arises from distal vertebral artery

supplies retro-olivary medulla, inferior vermis, tonsil, and inferior lateral posterior surface of cerebellar hemisphere

most frequent cause of PICA infarct is thrombosis of vertebral artery

anterior inferior cerebellar artery (AICA)

in equilibrium with PICA, the larger the PICA territory, the smaller the AICA territory (and vice versa)

supplies inferior lateral anterior surface of cerebellar hemisphere

superior cerebellar artery (SCA)

clinical presentation (infarction)—ipsilateral cerebellar ataxia, nausea, dysarthria (difficulty in articulation), and contralateral loss of pain and temperature sensation

supplies superior aspect of cerebellum, pons, and pineal gland

- imaging appearance

MR—more sensitive than CT for detecting acute ischemia in the major vascular territories (changes routinely noted by 4–6 hours post-ictus); marked superiority for detection of lacunar infarcts and for posterior fossa and brainstem lesions

infarct age

acute (day 0–7)—cytotoxic edema (abnormal accumulation of intracellular water—a shift of water from extra- to intracellular, with no net overall change), seen as early as 2 hours post-ictus

subtle narrowing of sulci and increase in thickness of gray mantle on T_1 (parenchymal swelling without signal abnormality)

no gross T_2 change

can be visualized directly by diffusion imaging

subacute (day 7–30)—vasogenic edema (increased extracellular water content)

low SI on T_1, high SI on T_2

chronic (>30 days in age)

cerebral atrophy—widened sulci, ex vacuo dilatation of ventricles

encephalomalacia (cystic changes)—CSF SI on all pulse sequences

gliosis—high SI on intermediate and heavily T_2-weighted scans, often surrounds encephalomalacic region

wallerian degeneration (a type of white matter atrophy)—anterograde degeneration of axons, secondary to injury of neuron

low SI on T_1, high SI on T_2, loss of tissue volume

often seen in corticospinal tract in old large infarcts involving motor cortex (posterior limb of internal capsule, cerebral peduncle, anterior pons, to anterior medulla—where fibers decussate)

enhancement patterns

intravascular enhancement—reflects slow arterial flow, timing—days 0–7 (earliest type of abnormal enhancement identified in infarction)

meningeal enhancement—adjacent to damaged tissue, uncommon, timing—days 1–3

parenchymal enhancement—gyriform in pattern, timing—usually not seen prior to 6 days, prominent in subacute infarction (7–30 days), may persist for up to 8 weeks

this pattern of enhancement permits differentiation of subacute infarction from chronic white matter ischemic changes

on occasion, a subacute infarct will be isointense on T_1 and T_2-weighted scans, with only parenchymal enhancement permitting identification

hemorrhage (MR more sensitive than CT)

petechial hemorrhage within gray matter (often following gyri) not uncommon in subacute infarction

T_1—high SI (methemoglobin, subacute blood)

T_2—often low SI (intracellular methemoglobin)

dystrophic calcification—can be seen in chronic infarcts (sometimes gyriform in pattern), may be visualized as slight hyperintensity on T_1

MRA can demonstrate

vessel occlusion and stenosis

pathways of collateral blood supply

lacunar infarcts

acute lesions best demonstrated on T_2 (due to edema, with high SI)

lesion enhancement (acute/subacute time period) consistently demonstrated following Gd chelate administration

IV-contrast injection important for lesion identification

(lesion seen on postcontrast scans only in 4 of 9 cases in one study)

infant—detection of ischemia requires special attention to imaging technique (use of TE $\geq$90 msec and TR $\geq$3500 msec for T_2, and TE $\leq$10 msec and TR $\leq$500 msec for T_1), due to increased normal brain-water content

CT

within first 48 hours after ictus, may be normal

angiography (film findings)

vessel occlusion or slow anterograde flow

retrograde flow

nonperfused areas

vascular blush ("luxury perfusion")

nonspecific findings

early draining veins

mass effect

ultrasound

superior to CT and MR in premature neonates for detection of ischemia; MR superior after 37 weeks gestational age

---

1.782

Hemorrhagic infarction

- general information

  on histologic exam, one-fifth of all infarcts are hemorrhagic

  hemorrhage occurs in ischemic brain which is reperfused

  predisposing conditions—lysis of embolus, opening of collaterals, restoration of normal blood pressure following hypotension, hypertension, anticoagulation

- imaging appearance

  MR (high-field)—capable of distinguishing acute, subacute, and chronic hemorrhagic infarcts (improved sensitivity to blood products with GRE sequences; poor sensitivity to blood products with low-magnetic field scanners)

  acute hemorrhagic infarction (hemorrhagic component)—isointense to slightly hypointense on T_1, hypointense on T_2 (deoxyhemoglobin)

  subacute hemorrhagic infarction—hyperintense on T_1, followed in time by hyperintensity on T_2 (methemoglobin)

  chronic hemorrhagic infarction—persistent hypointensity on T_2 (hemosiderin/ferritin)

1.79

Periventricular leukomalacia (PVL)

- infarction of periventricular white matter in premature infant
- clinical presentation

spastic diplegia, quadriplegia, cerebral palsy

cortical blindness

mental retardation (severe cases)

- pathogenesis

    occurs in infants <1500 g birth weight or <35 weeks gestational age with respiratory distress syndrome

    autoregulation of cerebral blood flow—not fully developed in immature brain

    PVL—result of white matter hypoperfusion in watershed areas

- imaging appearance

    ultrasound (early stages)

        increased periventricular echogenicity

    MR (late stages)

        decreased quantity of periventricular white matter, with abnormal increased SI on T_2 in that remaining (gliosis)

            areas most commonly affected—adjacent to trigone and frontal horn

        ventriculomegaly (ex vacuo)

        thinning of corpus callosum

Miscellaneous ....

1.821

Obstructive noncommunicating hydrocephalus

- acutely—fluid forced out of ventricles into adjacent white matter—due to increased pressure
- imaging appearance

    MR—transependymal resorption of CSF

        thick smooth rim of periventricular white matter hyperintensity on T_2

    differential diagnosis

        small vessel ischemic disease

        demyelinating diseases (MS)—patchy

        radiation white matter injury—scalloped laterally, extends to cortical gray matter

1.83

Alzheimer's disease

- clinical presentation

    the most common cause of dementia

- histologic appearance (nonspecific)

    neurofibrillary tangles

    neuritic (senile) plaques

Hirano bodies

granulovacuolar degeneration

- imaging appearance

generalized cerebral atrophy (gray matter loss)

accentuated temporal lobe atrophy

1.837

Small vessel ischemic disease

- pathogenesis

areas of necrosis, small infarcts, demyelination, astroglia proliferation, arteriolosclerosis

mechanism—ischemia—penetrating arterioles

- imaging appearance (MR >> CT)

foci of increased T_2 SI

subcortical white matter

periventricular white matter

centrum semiovale

"capping" of lateral ventricles

patchy, relatively symmetric (right vs. left) involvement

1.85

Fibrous dysplasia

- pathogenesis

developmental skeletal anomaly

monostotic form

involvement of skull or face in 10–25%

polyostotic form

with endocrine dysfunction (precocious puberty in girl) = McCune-Albright syndrome

involvement of skull or face in 50%

- imaging appearance

lesions are well vascularized, with small vessels in center and large sinusoids in periphery

plain film

lucent or sclerotic

hazy ("ground glass") lucent lesions—of skull—typically expansile (with widening of diploic space)

1.871

Multiple sclerosis (MS)

- clinical presentation

20–40 years of age

pediatric presentation—rare

higher incidence in women (2:1)

highest incidence in temperate zones (US, Canada, Great Britain, Northern Europe)

relapsing, remitting, with eventual progression

weakness, numbness of extremities

bladder dysfunction

optic neuritis

- disease classification (clinical criteria)

  McAlpine

  "definite" MS—characteristic transient neurologic symptoms, with one or more documented relapses

  "probable" MS—one or more attacks of disease, with clinical evidence in first attack of multiple lesions

  "possible" MS—similar history to "probable" disease, but with paucity of findings or unusual features

  Schumacher

  "clinically definite" MS—evidence of two or more separate CNS lesions (by history or exam), clinical evidence of white matter involvement, two episodes each more than 24 hours duration and separated in time by more than 1 month, age 10–50 (arbitrary age limits)

- imaging appearance

  MR—markedly superior to CT for lesion detection

  punctate white matter lesions

  chronic lesions—small

  active lesions—larger, with less well-defined margins, may evoke minimal vasogenic edema

  asymmetric involvement (right vs. left brain)

  predisposition for (characteristic areas of involvement)

  immediate periventricular white matter

  corpus callosum (involvement of white matter adjacent to CSF, with radiation from ventricular surface)

  callosal lesions best detected on sagittal imaging

  relatively specific for MS

  colliculi

  middle cerebellar peduncles

  pons, medulla

  rare presentation—solitary giant lesion (CT or MR)—mimicking primary neoplasm, metastatic disease, or infection

  plaques best visualized on intermediate T_2-weighted scans (lesions are high SI on T_2, low SI on T_1)

  lesions adjacent to CSF obscured by high SI of CSF on heavily T_2-weighted scans

  absence of detected lesions (brain) does not rule out diagnosis

  with high suspicion of disease, examination of spinal cord by MR recommended lesion detection improved by use of thin sections (3–4 mm slice thickness)

acquisition of both sagittal and axial sections recommended

nonspecific findings (chronic disease)

ventricular enlargement

cerebral atrophy

thinning of corpus callosum

contrast enhancement

majority of lesions visualized are chronic in nature, do not demonstrate enhancement

lesion enhancement best seen on early postcontrast (vs. delayed) scans

lesion enhancement is transient, exists for <4 weeks in most cases, correlates with active disease, a marker for new lesions

both punctate and ring enhancement occur

disease severity

in early MS, few plaques may be seen

in severe, late involvement, periventricular plaques may become confluent

- differential diagnosis

ischemic and gliottic white matter lesions (small vessel ischemic disease)

such lesions tend to be symmetrical in distribution (right vs. left brain), and are often confluent

neurosarcoidosis

SLE (usually not periventricular)

acute disseminated encephalomyelitis (ADEM)

1.872

Acute disseminated encephalomyelitis (ADEM)

- clinical presentation

children, following viral illness (measles) or vaccination (rabies, tetanus)

confusion, somnolence, coma (severe cases), convulsions, headache, fever, ataxia

monophasic

- pathogenesis

inflammatory and demyelinating disease of white matter (perivenular)

- imaging appearance

MR

white matter lesions, peripheral and deep in location, typically ill-defined margins

cerebrum, cerebellum, brainstem

enhancement—common in acute presentation—with majority of lesions demonstrating enhancement

lesion resolution can be noted with successful treatment (high-dose steroids)

CT

despite severe disease, scan can be normal

MR >> CT for lesion detection

1.873

Adrenoleukodystrophy (ADL)

- clinical presentation

    adrenal insufficiency

    progressive multifocal CNS demyelination

- pathogenesis

    childhood ADL

        most common form of X-linked ADL

        defective gene—in Xq28 region of X chromosome

        impaired degradation of saturated very long-chain fatty acids

        onset at 5–14 years of age, with rapid neurologic deterioration

- imaging appearance

    MR/CT

        involvement of splenium of corpus callosum, fornix, parieto-occipital white matter (low SI on T_1, high SI on T_2, low attenuation on CT)

        posterior to anterior disease progression

        atypical patterns of white matter disease have been described, specifically frontal, cerebellar, and asymmetrical involvement

        can demonstrate mild enhancement along anterior margin (leading edge) of involved white matter

Canavan's disease

- clinical presentation—first 6 months of life

    macrocephaly (the other leukodystrophy with this finding is Alexander's disease)

    hypotonia

    developmental regression

    cortical blindness

- pathogenesis

    autosomal recessive

    deficiency of enzyme aspartoacylase

- imaging appearance (nonspecific)

    MR/CT

        cortical atrophy

        ventriculomegaly

symmetric abnormal white matter (high SI on T$_2$)—as with most of the leukodystrophies

Leigh's disease

- clinical presentation
  - infants/children
  - feeding difficulties
  - psychomotor retardation
  - visual disturbances
- pathogenesis
  - autosomal recessive
  - cerebral inhibition of ATP-TPP (adenosine 5'-triphosphate-thiamine pyrophosphate) phosphoryltransferase
- imaging appearance
  - MR—abnormal high SI on T$_2$ in
    - spinal cord
    - brainstem
    - basal ganglia (putamen)
    - optic pathways

Other inherited metabolic (storage) diseases—on imaging—cerebral atrophy, or diffuse white matter abnormality

- lipidoses
  - Gaucher's disease
  - Niemann-Pick disease
  - Krabbe's disease
  - Fabry's disease
  - G$_{M1}$ gangliosidosis
  - G$_{M2}$ gangliosidosis (Tay-Sachs disease)
- mucopolysaccharidoses
  - Hurler's disease
  - Hunter's disease
  - Scheie's disease
  - Sanfilippo's disease
  - Morquio's disease
- mucolipidoses
- glycogenoses

1.879

Central pontine myelinolysis

- clinical presentation
  - flaccid quadriplegia
  - facial, pharyngeal, glottic paralysis

- pathogenesis

    osmotic injury, secondary to rapid correction of severe chronic hyponatremia (alcoholism, malnutrition)

    symmetric destruction of myelin sheaths—starting at median raphe of pons

- imaging appearance

    CT

    usually negative

    MR

    abnormal high T_2 SI—pons, middle cerebellar peduncles

    differential diagnosis—infarction, metastasis, glioma, MS, radiation changes

---

1.882, 1.883

Cerebellar degenerative disease

- alcoholic

    atrophy and degeneration of cerebellar vermis and hemispheres—occurs in up to 40% of chronic alcoholics

    irreversible

    clinical presentation

    broad-based staggering gait

    truncal instability

    ataxia

    impaired heel-to-toe walking

    pathogenesis

    direct toxic effects of alcohol

    thiamine deficiency

- primary forms

    differentiated by olivary atrophy, which is not present in alcoholism

    olivopontocerebellar degeneration

    atrophy of the pons, middle cerebellar peduncles, inferior olivary nuclei and cerebellar hemispheres

    clinical presentation—ataxia, first in lower, then in upper extremities

    imaging appearance—atrophy, gliosis

    cerebello-olivary degeneration

1.884

Huntington's disease

- MR > CT for demonstration of morphologic changes

    thin section heavily T_1- or T_2-weighted imaging recommended

- clinical presentation

    fourth to sixth decades

           choreoathetosis

           progressive dementia

- pathogenesis

           autosomal dominant inheritance (chromosome 4)

           premature death of certain neurons

- imaging appearance

           degeneration, volume loss—corpus striatum (caudate nucleus, putamen)

           cortical atrophy—in longstanding disease

HEAD AND NECK

Base of Skull ....

Central Skull Base

- bones of skull base—derived from cartilage (vs. cranial vault—formed by membranous ossification)
- spheno-occipital synchondrosis (in clivus)—last to fuse (age 25)

12.11

Normal anatomy

- sphenoid bone
    - foundation of central skull base
    - forms floor of middle cranial fossa, cavernous sinus, pituitary gland
    - shape—birdlike with outstretched wings—central body, two sets of wings (greater, lesser), medial and lateral pterygoid plates (inferiorly)
- basal foramina
    - foramen rotundum
        - located medially in anterior greater wing
        - contains maxillary nerve (V_2)
    - foramen ovale
        - located in floor of middle cranial fossa
        - contains mandibular nerve (V_3)
    - foramen spinosum
        - located posterolateral to foramen ovale
        - contains middle meningeal artery, meningeal branch of mandibular nerve
    - foramen lacerum (not really a foramen)
        - located at base of medial pterygoid plate
    - pterygoid (vidian) canal
        - located at base of pterygoid plates, medial and below foramen rotundum
        - contains vidian artery and nerve
- pituitary gland
    - covered by dura—diaphragma sella
    - two main parts
        - anterior pituitary (adenohypophysis)—pars anterior and pars intermedia (separated by cleft—in which embryologic remnants may be present—Rathke's cleft cyst)
        - posterior pituitary (neurohypophysis)
- cavernous sinus
    - borders pituitary gland on each side
    - contains internal carotid artery, with abducens nerve laterally (VI)
    - contains laterally (from superior to inferior)—oculomotor nerve (III), trochlear nerve (IV), ophthalmic (V_1) and maxillary (V_2) divisions of trigeminal nerve

tributaries—superior ophthalmic veins, sphenoparietal sinus

drainage—superior and inferior petrosal sinuses

- clivus

  portion of skull base between dorsum sellae and foramen magnum—includes body of sphenoid bone and basioccipital portion of occipital bone

---

12.1211

CT technique

- axial (parallel to Reid's base line—line from infraorbital rim to external auditory canal) and coronal sections (perpendicular to Reid's base line); 1.5–3-mm slice thickness
- if problems encountered in coronal cuts due to dental amalgam—use less tilt or reconstruct from thin section axials
- for bone detail—use high resolution bone algorithm with wide windows
- for soft tissue evaluation—IV contrast necessary

12.1214

MR technique

- coil—use that standard for head
- sagittal (primarily for localization) and axial (T_2 and T_1) and coronal (T_1) planes; 3-mm slice thickness
- IV contrast necessary

12.14

Congenital/Developmental abnormalities

- arachnoid cyst

  contains CSF

  may expand with time

  may cause bony changes—thinning, elevation of lesser wing, anterior displacement of greater wing

  middle cranial fossa—most common location

- cephalocele

  protrusion of cranial contents through congenital defect

  meningocele—contains meninges and subarachnoid space

  encephalocele—also contains brain

  midline (vertex or skull base)—most common location

  encephaloceles—incidence by location—10% at skull base (sphenopharyngeal = sincipital is most common basal type—presents with airway obstruction, CSF leak, meningitis; other types—spheno-orbital, sphenoethmoidal; transethmoidal); 75% occipital in location; 15% at nose/orbit

  CT—defines bony defect

  MR—identifies presence/absence of brain tissue

- craniosynostosis = premature fusion

    cranial sutures normally begin to fuse at age 3 and are completely fused by age 6

    premature fusion—prevents normal brain development

12.3

Neoplasm, neoplasticlike condition

- benign tumors

    juvenile angiofibroma

    highly vascular, locally invasive (highly aggressive)

    location—nasopharynx

    clinical presentation—nasal obstruction, epistaxis, adolescent males

    spread beyond nasopharynx at presentation common—usually via pterygopalatine fossa into infratemporal fossa

    MR—vascular flow voids may be seen

    meningioma

    skull base—one third of all meningiomas

    locations

    sphenoid wing (most)—includes hyperostosing en plaque type and those involving clinoid (latter can extend into cavernous sinus)

    olfactory groove

    tuberculum sellae

    pituitary tumors

    benign adenomas (majority of lesions)—from adenohypophyseal cells

    slow-growing, histologically benign

    microadenoma—<1 cm; macroadenoma—>1 cm

    characterized by endocrine features—most are prolactin-secreting

- malignant tumors

    Chondrosarcoma

    spread by local invasion, recurrence common

    calcification of tumor matrix—hallmark

    erode, destroy bone

    common locations—parasellar, cerebellopontine (CP) angle, along convexity

    chordoma

    arise from remnants of embryonic notochord

    one third in skull base—clivus, spheno-occipital synchondrosis

    peak incidence—age 20–40 (vs. 40–60 for sacrococcygeal chordomas)

    slow-growing, poor prognosis—infiltrative, almost 100% recurrence bone destruction, soft tissue mass—commonly with calcification or bone fragments

MR better than CT for delineation

nasopharyngeal carcinoma

high incidence in Chinese

often asymptomatic, with delayed diagnosis

spread by local infiltration

rhabdomyosarcoma

most common soft tissue sarcoma of children

peak incidence—age 2–5

location—most in head and neck (one third pharynx)

skull base invasion—poor prognosis

metastatic disease

infrequent to skull base, but more common than primary bone lesions

common primaries—prostate, lung, breast

- miscellaneous

Paget's disease

about one half with skull involvement—bony thickening and sclerosis most common appearance in skull base

fibrous dysplasia

skull base commonly involved with polyostotic disease

lesion may be pagetoid, sclerotic, or cystic in appearance

12.4

Trauma

- fractures

most in skull base are extensions of cranial vault fractures

clinical presentation—CSF otorrhea/rhinorrhea, hemotympanum, mastoid region ecchymosis, cranial nerve deficits

CT—axial, thin section—method of choice for examination

- CSF fistula

most common cause—trauma

high risk of infection

CT cisternography—method of choice (has replaced radioisotope studies since site of injury is more accurately demonstrated)

Congenital Lesions ....

2.1461 and 2.1462

Cephalocele

- congenital herniation of intracranial contents through defect in cranium

meningocele—contains only meninges

encephalocele—also contains brain

- classification—by site of defect

  occipital—most frequent (>50%)

  cranial vault

  frontoethmoidal (sincipital)—visible externally—most frequent type in certain Southeast Asian groups

      nasofrontal

      nasoethmoidal

      naso-orbital

  basal—not visible externally—frequently associated with generalized craniofacial/craniocerebral dysraphism

      transethmoidal

      sphenoethmoidal

      transphenoidal

      frontosphenoidal

2.1463

Nasal dermal sinus/cyst

- sinus = small epithelial-lined tube, extending from skin surface (along midline of nose) to variable depth (may reach intradural space)

  treatment—surgical resection (cosmetic/prevention of meningitis)

- cyst = midline epithelial-lined cyst lying along expected course of dermal sinus; may be either a dermoid or an epidermoid (equally common)
- imaging—CT—displays well sinus tract, bony channels, infection

---

2.1469

Nasal glioma (very uncommon)

- benign glial tissue mass of congenital origin
- occurs intranasally or extranasally at root of nose
- may be connected by pedicle of glial tissue to brain
- does not contain CSF

2.148

Cleft lip, palate, face

- common (lateral) cleft lip

  nasomedial and maxillary processes fail to merge

  unilateral or bilateral

- common (lateral) cleft palate

  posterior extension to include palate

  unilateral or bilateral

- midline cleft lip (inferior group)—rare

  cleft involves upper lip (with/without nose)

  associated findings—hypertelorism, basal encephaloceles, callosal agenesis, optic nerve dysplasias

- median cleft face (superior group) = frontonasal dysplasia—rare
  cleft involves nose (with/without forehead/upper lip)
  associated findings—hypertelorism, broad nasal root, cranium bifidum, frontonasal/intraorbital encephaloceles, callosal lipomas, anophthalmos/microphthalmos

Temporal Bone ....

21.11

Normal anatomy

- temporal bone (divided into five parts, listed below):
  1. squamous—anterolateral, upper part of temporal bone
     thin, shell-like
     attachment of temporalis muscle
     wall for part of temporal fossa zygomatic process—arises from lower portion, arches anteriorly (medial surface—origin of masseter muscle)
  2. mastoid—in adult, continues inferiorly as mastoid process—attachment for sternocleidomastoid, splenius capitis, longissimus capitis, and digastric muscles
     contains tympanic antrum (large irregular cavity, in upper, anterior part of mastoid) which communicates with mastoid air cells and epitympanum (attic) via a small canal (aditus ad antrum)
  3. petrous—at base of skull between sphenoid bone anteriorly and occipital bone posteriorly
     contains inner ear
     opening of internal auditory canal (IAC) = porus acusticus
     fundus of IAC
        divided into upper and lower compartments by bony crest = crista falciformis
        upper compartment—contains facial nerve (VII) anteriorly and superior vestibular division of VIII posteriorly
        lower compartment—cochlear division of VIII anteriorly and inferior vestibular division of VIII posteriorly
     jugular foramen—has two compartments
        pars nervosa (medial)—contains inferior petrosal sinus, glossopharyngeal nerve (IX)
        pars vascularis (lateral)—contains internal jugular vein, vagus nerve (X) and spinal accessory nerve (XI)
  4. tympanic—curved plate below squamous section and anterior to mastoid
  5. styloid process—projects down and anterior from undersurface of temporal bone, just anterior to stylomastoid foramen
- external auditory canal
- middle ear (tympanic cavity)—air-filled (via eustachian tube), traversed by auditory ossicles (which connect lateral and medial walls); three parts —tympanic cavity proper (next to tympanic membrane), attic/

epitympanum (above membrane), hypotympanum (below membrane); shaped like a cleft

roof (tegmental wall)—separates middle ear from middle cranial fossa

floor (jugular wall)—separates middle ear from internal jugular vein

mastoid (posterior) wall—contains entrance to tympanic antrum (aditus ad antrum)

carotid (anterior) wall

Eustachian tube—connection between nasopharynx and tympanic cavity

lateral (membranous) wall = tympanic membrane—manubrium of malleus is attached at center medially

medial (labyrinthine) wall—separates middle and inner ears, contains oval and round windows

epitympanic recess = attic = that part of cavity above tympanic membrane

contains head of malleus and incus

contents of tympanic cavity

ossicles—malleus, incus, stapes (lateral to medial)

muscles—tensor tympani and stapedius—act to reduce efficiency of sound conduction

- facial nerve (cranial nerve VII)—motor (larger) and sensory roots

motor root

intracranial segment—medulla to porus acusticus

IAC segment

labyrinthine segment—when just lateral and superior to cochlea, angles forward to reach geniculate ganglion

tympanic segment—turns posteriorly (first genu)

mastoid segment—turns vertically (second genu)

- inner ear

bony labyrinth

vestibule— arge ovoid perilymphatic space (connects anteriorly to cochlea, posteriorly to semicircular canals)

semicircular canals—superior, lateral (horizontal), and posterior

cochlea—like a cone, with apex pointing anteriorly, laterally, and slightly down; two-and-a-half to two-and-three-fourths turns

membranous labyrinth—interconnecting spaces form endolymphatic cavity

21.1211

CT technique

- depicts bony detail
- 1.5 mm sections; axial—with chin slightly extended, bone detail software; coronal—performed as an adjunct
- IV contrast—for hypervascular lesions (glomus tumor), cerebellopontine angle (CPA) masses, lesion extension intracranially or below skull base

21.1214

MR technique

- depicts soft tissue and fluid-containing structures
- 3-mm axial and coronal sections
- IV contrast—for question of neoplasia or inflammation/infection

21.14

Congenital anomalies

- outer ear
  - stenosis of external auditory canal—can develop acquired cholesteatoma
  - atresia of external auditory canal—may have congenital cholesteatoma of middle ear
- middle ear
  - tympanic ring dysplasia
  - tympanic ring aplasia (bony plate takes place of tympanic membrane and external auditory canal)—common with thalidomide; fusion of malleus to atretic plate
- inner ear
  - bony labyrinth
  - membranous labyrinth
- vascular
  - high jugular bulb
    - thin bony covering
    - bulb vulnerable to trauma
  - protruding jugular bulb (protrudes into middle ear)
    - dehiscence of middle ear floor
- malformations associated with meningitis (due to CSF leak)
  - IAC—defect in lamina cribrosa which separates IAC and vestibule
  - dehiscence of tegmen tympani (roof of middle ear)
  - wide cochlear aqueduct

21.2

Inflammation

- middle ear effusion
  - in adult, must rule out (r/o) obstructing neoplasm in nasopharynx
- mastoiditis
  - CT (nonspecific appearance)—patchy opacification of multiple mastoid air cells
  - complications (inadequate treatment)
    - demineralization of trabeculae, with eventual formation of one large cavity

sixth nerve palsy, fifth nerve pain (involvement of petrous apex)

sigmoid sinus thrombosis, meningitis, abscess (all possible if disruption of mastoid cortex occurs)

- granulation tissue

  common

  subtype—cholesterol granuloma

    smooth, erosive mass

    high SI on T_1 (hemorrhage)

- cholesteatoma (acquired)

  enlarging sac of stratified squamous epithelium containing exfoliated keratin

  vast majority in temporal bone (middle ear) are acquired (secondary to tympanic membrane defects)

  cause bony destruction

    potential complication—labyrinthine fistula (most due to erosion in region of lateral semicircular canal)

- conductive deafness—high incidence with cholesteatoma (due to ossicular erosions) and also in noncholesteatomatous chronic otitis media (due to ossicular erosions or fixation)

- postoperative—CT is the exam of choice—need to examine/describe following:

  surgical defect

  residual debris (recurrent cholesteatoma, granulation tissue, and surgical packing cannot be differentiated)

  bony defects (especially those in roof = tegmen or floor = jugular wall)

  ossicular chain

    Proplast or Plastopore used for total or partial ossicular replacement

    cochlear implants (for profound sensorineural deafness)—electrode stimulates cochlea

  exclude fistula

  facial nerve canal

- otitis externa (involvement of external auditory canal)—can be life-threatening in diabetic or immunocompromised patient

---

21.31

Neoplasm (temporal bone, CPA)

- MR and/or CT indicated
- acoustic schwannoma (neuroma)

  10% of intracranial tumors, majority of CPA tumors

  clinical presentation—age 30–70, more common in women; neurofibromatosis 2—>95% have bilateral acoustic schwannomas, present earlier than unilateral lesions; symptoms—sensorineural hearing loss, tinnitus, disequilibrium

  pathology—benign, slow-growing, encapsulated; arise within IAC or at porus acusticus; variable growth rates

CT

majority of medium-sized lesions have spherical component in cistern (centered on porus) with stem extending into and expanding IAC

small percent entirely intracanalicular, with cylindrical shape

enhancement in >90% (homogeneous, dense)

MR

superior to CT for detection of small lesions

intense enhancement

when large—displace, deform brainstem

other tumors of CPA (in order of incidence)—meningioma (3%), epidermoid (2%), other (1%) cranial nerve neuromas (V, VII, IX, X, XI)

- meningioma

differentiating features from acoustic schwannoma

usually eccentric to porus acusticus

frequently herniate into middle cranial fossa

broad-based against dural surface—hemispherical in shape (vs. spherical for acoustic schwannoma)

form obtuse angle (between tumor and bone)—vs. acute angle for acoustic schwannoma

often calcified

- epidermoid (= primary cholesteatoma = pearly tumor)

congenital, but do not appear until adulthood

composition—stratified squamous epithelial surrounding desquamated keratin

very slow growth (reach considerable size with minimal symptoms)

variable shape, nonenhancing

CT—CSF density

MR—slightly hyperintense to CSF on T_1- and intermediate T_2-weighted images

- other cranial nerve neuromas

resemble acoustic schwannomas in appearance, but not location

trigeminal—most common

can involve both posterior and middle cranial fossae

can extend into Meckel's cave

more prone to cystic components than acoustic schwannoma

- vascular lesions

vertebrobasilar dolichoectasia—can cause compression of cranial nerves (facial and trigeminal most common)

definition

elongation—if basilar artery is lateral to clivus or bifurcation is above plane of suprasellar cistern

ectasia—diameter of basilar artery >4.5 mm (by CT)

vascular loop (anterior inferior cerebellar artery [AICA])—vertigo

AICA aneurysm—acoustic or facial nerve symptoms

pial (superficial) siderosis of acoustic nerve—from recurrent hemorrhage

- paraganglioma (glomus tumors)

  terminology (location)

      glomus tympanicum—tympanic cavity and mastoid

      glomus jugulare—jugular bulb and skull base

      glomus vagale—parapharyngeal

  clinical presentation

      three times more common in women

      fourth and fifth decades

      may be bilateral

      other tumors, such as carotid body, may be present

      otologic symptoms (hearing loss, tinnitus) predominate for both tympanicum and jugulare tumors

  pathology

      locally infiltrating

      slow growth

      can be lethal if not treated

  imaging appearance

      CT—useful for planning surgical approach (bony landmarks)

          localized bone destruction common

          grow along path of least resistance

          glomus tympanicum—present early, well-defined soft tissue mass, no bone involvement; as growth occurs involve jugular fossa (spread from hypotympanum through jugular wall)

          important differential diagnosis—aberrant carotid artery or exposed jugular bulb—can present to otologist with symptoms similar to paraganglioma

      MR—useful for localization and differential diagnosis

          salt and pepper appearance (mixed hyper- and hypointensity) on both T_1 and T_2

          flow voids

      angiography—useful for differential diagnosis and preoperative embolization (specifically for glomus jugulare tumors, which can have high blood loss)

          hypervascular (characteristic)

          enlarged feeding arteries, with rapid venous drainage

          feeding vessels common from ascending pharyngeal artery

  treatment—resection ("cure") or radiation (to control growth)

- other jugular foramen tumors—10% of masses in jugular foramen are not glomus tumors

  differential diagnosis (common lesions)

      schwannoma (jugular fossa or hypoglossal)

      meningioma

- tumors involving facial nerve—only 6% of facial nerve disorders (>50% = Bell's palsy)

schwannoma—can occur anywhere along length of nerve

clinical presentation—compress, do not invade nerve, thus may not have facial palsy; present with hearing loss

imaging appearance—variable size, may be quite large

hemangioma, vascular malformations

epidermoid (congenital or primary cholesteatoma)—can arise in both intradural and extradural (petrous apex, supralabyrinthine) locations

CT—bone margins characteristically sharp

- tumors of external auditory canal

squamous cell carcinoma—most common malignant tumor

- other lesions of petrous apex—beware of pitfall—asymmetrical pneumatization or unilateral retention of secretions in air cells of petrous apex can be mistaken for tumor on MR

cholesterol granuloma (cyst)—contains cholesterol and blood products (high SI on T_1 and T_2); treated by surgical drainage

epidermoid—much less common in petrous apex than cholesterol granuloma; treated by surgical excision

carotid artery aneurysm

chondrosarcoma—causes bone destruction, may contain calcifications, enhances postcontrast; locally invasive

---

21.4

Trauma

- fracture types

longitudinal (in long axis of temporal bone)

result of blow to temporoparietal area

ossicular derangement and tympanic membrane perforation common

increased long-term risk of cholesteatoma

transverse

result of blow to frontal or occipital area

involvement of labyrinth (acute hearing loss, severe vertigo) common

mixed (majority)

- detailed inspection of course of facial nerve (in cases of paralysis) important (early surgery indicated for impingement)
- disruption of tegmen tympani—cause of CSF otorrhea

21.87

Otosclerosis

- resorption of normal endochondral layer, with deposition of new spongy vascular bone
- high incidence of bilateral disease

clinical presentation—hearing loss

- CT—active phase—demineralization; chronic phase—sclerosis

Orbit ....

22.11

Orbit proper—Normal anatomy

- bone
    - orbital apex
        - optic canal—contains optic nerve, ophthalmic artery
        - superior orbital fissure—inferolateral to optic canal; contains oculomotor, trochlear, abducens nerves, branches of ophthalmic nerve, ophthalmic veins
    - inferior orbital fissure—contains maxillary nerve
    - periosteum of bony orbit = periorbita—posteriorly contiguous with dura around optic nerve, surgery/trauma can lead to CSF leaks posteriorly
    - medial wall—lamina papyracea (paper thin)
    - bony interorbital distance (BID)—with CT, can be measured at any desired point (vs. plain film)—one standard is measurement at posterior border of frontal processes of maxillae
- soft tissues
    - extraocular muscles
        - superior rectus
        - inferior rectus
        - medial rectus
        - lateral rectus
        - superior oblique—longest and thinnest, passes anteriorly and medially through trochlea turning posteriolaterally and downward to insert on lateral sclera
        - inferior oblique—only muscle not to originate from orbital apex; originates from maxilla
        - levator palpebrae—between superior rectus muscle and roof of orbit; may not be possible to separate from superior rectus muscle on CT/MR
    - intraconal space—separated from other spaces (conal, extraconal) by rectus muscles
    - lacrimal gland
        - location—superolateral in orbit
        - vascular supply—lacrimal artery, superior ophthalmic vein
        - tears produced by gland pass across cornea and are absorbed through lacrimal canaliculi of upper and lower lids
- innervation
    - III (oculomotor)—supplies superior, inferior, medial recti, inferior oblique, levator palpebrae
    - IV (trochlea)—supplies superior oblique muscle
    - VI (abducens)—supplies lateral rectus muscle
- vascular anatomy
    - arterial supply—ophthalmic artery

venous drainage—superior (empties into cavernous sinus) and inferior (smaller, variable) ophthalmic veins

---

22.1211

Orbit—CT technique

- axial and coronal sections; 5-mm slice thickness (3 mm for exam of optic nerve, 1.5 mm to detect foreign bodies or for exam of globe)—axial exam should be obtained parallel to infraorbital-meatal line
- 0.05 Gy/slice dose to lens
- for evaluation of lesion vascularity—IV contrast necessary

22.1214

Orbit—MR technique

- coil—use that standard for head
- axial (T_2 and T_1); ≤5-mm slice thickness; supplemental sagittal/coronal for optic nerve lesions
- fat suppression (short tau inversion recovery [STIR] or spectral presaturation)
- IV contrast—tumors, optic nerve lesions, orbital masses

22.143

Orbit, anomalies, definitions

- hypertelorism—medial walls of orbits further apart than normal (eyes usually widely spaced) = increased BID
- hypotelorism—decreased BID (eyes usually appear too close or normally spaced)
- exophthalmos—prominence of globe (proptosis—protrusion of globe)
- exorbitism—decrease in volume of orbit (orbit contents, globe protrude)
- craniosynostosis (craniostenosis)—premature closure of one or more sutures—orbital abnormalities are primarily from coronal synostosis
  premature suture closures/result
  > metopic/trigonocephaly (triangular head)
  > sagittal/scaphocephaly (dolichocephaly)
  > unilateral coronal or lambdoid/plagiocephaly
  >> bilateral coronal or lambdoid/brachycephaly

22.2

Orbit, inflammation

- infection—majority of primary orbital disease, usually of sinus origin
- orbital cellulitis—stages in evolution from sinusitis:
  1. inflammatory edema (preseptal cellulitis)—infection still confined to paranasal sinus, edema due to venous congestion

    2. subperiosteal phlegmon, abscess

    3. orbital cellulitis (infiltration of periorbital and retro-orbital fat)

    4. orbital abscess

    5. ophthalmic vein, cavernous sinus thrombosis

- mycotic infection

    mucormycosis (rhinocerebral form)

    aspergillosis

- orbital pseudotumor—encompasses broad category of orbital inflammatory disease

    definition—idiopathic inflammation, without identifiable cause or systemic disease

        many cases with time turn out to be malignant lymphoma

    types

        anterior orbital inflammation

        diffuse orbital pseudotumor—does not distort globe (or intraorbital contents) nor invade bone; difficult to differentiate from lymphoma

        orbital myositis—one or more extraocular muscles involved; major differential diagnosis is Graves' disease

        apical orbital inflammation

        lacrimal adenitis

        perineuritis

    CT—demonstrates contrast enhancement (lymphoma does not), infiltration of retrobulbar fat, no edema of eyelids

- thyroid disease

    unilateral or bilateral, when bilateral usually symmetric

    inferior rectus muscle most commonly involved (with limitation of elevation of affected eye)

    enlargement of muscle belly, with sparing of tendon

- sarcoidosis—most common type of involvement of orbit is chronic lacrimal adenitis

---

22.3

Orbit, neoplasm

22.34   Leukemia, lymphoma

- lymphoma

    continuum from benign to malignant—which cannot be differentiated by imaging

    75% have systemic lymphoma

    CT/MR—homogeneous, sharp margins, does not erode bone nor enlarge orbit (lesion molds itself around structures), mild enhancement

- leukemia—infiltration of bone or soft tissue by leukemic cells

22.36 Benign soft tissue neoplasm

- hemangioma
    capillary—infants in first year of life, most common location—superior nasal quadrant, usually involute by 1 year of age
    cavernous—most common vascular orbital tumor in adult age—second to fourth decades
        slow progressive enlargement
        fibrous pseudocapsule—appears well-defined on imaging
        most frequently occur in retrobulbar muscle cone
        CT/MR—smoothly marginated, homogeneous, lobulated, variable enhancement, orbital bone expansion not uncommon
- lymphangioma
    gradually enlarge with time (vs. capillary hemangioma)
    composed of lymph-filled sinuses
    typically not well-encapsulated (poorly circumscribed), thus can infiltrate normal tissues
    recurrence common
- orbital varix—CT should be performed with patient prone and during Valsalva maneuver
- carotid-cavernous fistula
    clinical presentation—proptosis, venous engorgement (superior ophthalmic vein), pulsating exophthalmos, bruit
    cause—trauma, surgery, or spontaneous
- schwannoma
    benign, slow-growing, nerve sheath tumor
    most common in intraconal space
    occur as isolated lesions or with neurofibromatosis
    CT/MR—sharply marginated, oval, fusiform, moderate-to-marked enhancement
- benign mixed tumor (pleomorphic adenoma)—lacrimal gland
    good prognosis if surgically removed en bloc without incisional biopsy (to ensure complete removal)
    well-encapsulated, round, long duration
    can indent globe, distort muscle cone, manifest bony destruction (unlike lymphoid/inflammatory processes)

22.26

Orbit, vasculitides—immune-complex mediated

- Wegener's granulomatosis—orbital involvement in one-fifth
- idiopathic midline destructive granuloma = lethal midline granuloma
- painful external ophthalmoplegia = Tolosa-Hunt syndrome
    idiopathic inflammatory process
    variant of pseudotumor
    responsive to corticosteroids

223

Tear duct system

- dacryocystography—used in evaluation of epiphora (overflow of tears on cheek)

    determines patency of canaliculi (upper and lower punctum to lacrimal sac), lacrimal sac, and nasolacrimal duct

    can diagnose obstruction (site and degree—most obstructions are complete and occur at junction of lacrimal sac and nasolacrimal duct), fistulae and diverticula (usually result of chronic obstruction), concretions

    radiographic technique

    > contrast material—water-soluble iodinated agent

    > cannula placed in lower punctum (lower lid, medial)

224.11

Eyeball—Normal anatomy

- posterior segment—vitreous chamber
- anterior segment—contains aqueous fluid produced by ciliary body
- Tenon's capsule—covers sclera, is a fibroelastic membrane, encloses posterior four-fifths of eyeball; tendons of extrinsic ocular muscles pierce capsule to reach sclera
- three primary layers

    sclera (outer layer)—collagen-elastic tissue

    uvea (middle layer)—vascular, contains iris, ciliary body, choroid; choroid divided into four layers: from internal to external Bruch's membrane, choriocapillaris (capillary layer), choroidal stroma, suprachoroidea; function of uvea—vascular supply to eye and regulation of ocular temperature

    retina (inner layer)—neural, sensory layer; inner layer—sensory retina; outer layer—retinal pigment epithelium (RPE); three potential spaces (thus detachments)—posterior hyaloid space (between base of hyaloid and sensory retina = posterior hyaloid detachment), subretinal space (between sensory retina and RPE = retinal detachment), suprachoroidal space (between choroid and sclera)

224.1211

Eyeball—CT technique

- 1.5–3-mm axial sections
- for foreign bodies and lesions at 6:00 or 12:00—need additional coronal sections

224.1214

Eyeball—MR technique

- obtain both head coil and surface coil images

- head coil images may at times be superior—due to SNR (thicker sections) and less motion artifact
- contraindicated in trauma with suspicion of ferromagnetic foreign body

---

224.3

Eyeball—neoplasm, neoplastic-like disease

- leukocoria—white or pink-white or yellow-white pupillary reflex; caused by reflection of incident light back through pupil; due to mass, membrane, detachment, or storage disease

  differential diagnosis—retinoblastoma, persistent hyperplastic primary vitreous (PHPV), retinopathy of prematurity (ROP), congenital cataract, Coats' disease, toxocariasis, retinal detachment

  most common presenting sign of retinoblastoma
- retinoblastoma

  most common childhood intraocular tumor (98% of cases present before 6 months of age)

  tumor is congenital, but usually not recognized at birth

  bilateral in 25% (these are hereditary)

  trilateral retinoblastoma—association of retinoblastoma and pinealoma

  growth may be endophytic, exophytic (can stimulate traumatic retinal detachment), or diffuse

  imaging—to determine retrobulbar spread, intracranial metastases, additional lesions

  CT—>90% show calcification (very few simulating lesions contain calcification)

  MR—not as specific as CT (poor sensitivity to calcification); T_1—slight-to-moderate high SI (vs. vitreous), T_2—marked-to-moderate low SI

  differential diagnosis—when total retinal detachment is present, other considerations include PHPV, Coats' disease, and ROP
- persistent hyperplastic primary vitreous (PHPV)

  heterogeneous etiology—congenital defect or systemic involvement

  clinically—usually unilateral leukocoria, microphthalmos, lens opacity, retinal detachment, vitreous hemorrhage

  best diagnosis—by demonstration of remnants of fetal hyaloid vascular system

  CT—enhancement of abnormal intravitreal tissue, presence of intravitreal tissue suggesting persistence of fetal tissue or congenital nonattachment of retina

  MR—marked hyperintensity of vitreous on T_1, proton density and T_2 (thus differentiated from retinoblastoma—hypointense vitreous on T_2); retinal detachment—2 types, from optic nerve vs. from point of wall eccentric to optic nerve
- Norrie's disease

  congenital progressive oculo-acoustic-cerebral degeneration

  X-linked recessive

retinal malformation, deafness, mental retardation/deterioration

CT—bilateral dense vitreous, retrolental mass, retinal detachment, optic nerve atrophy, microphthalmia

MR—bilateral hyperintense vitreous due to hemorrhage

- Warburg's syndrome

    hydrocephalus, agyria, retinal dysplasia/detachment

    congenital

    imaging—bilateral retinal detachment, vitreous and subretinal hemorrhage

- retinopathy of prematurity (ROP)

    usually due to prolonged exposure to supplemental oxygen

    retinal neovascularization, detachment, leaving a dense retrolental membrane and microphthalmus

- Coats' disease

    idiopathic retinal telangiectasis, breakdown of blood-retinal barrier, and exudative retinal detachment

    unilateral

    can resemble retinoblastoma on ophthalmoscopic exam

    CT—cannot distinguish Coats' from unilateral retinoblastoma without calcification

    MR—subretinal exudation is hyperintense on all sequences, vs. retinoblastoma which is hypointense on T_2

- ocular toxocariasis

    infection due to ingestion of eggs of *Toxocara canis*

    chronic retinal detachment, organized vitreous

    CT—diffuse or locally thickened uveosclera

- coloboma

    a notch or hole with tissue missing, congenital or acquired

    coloboma of optic nerve—one cause of leukocoria

    CT/MR—posterior globe defect with optic disc excavation, can have colobomatous cyst

- malignant uveal melanoma

    most common primary or metastatic ocular neoplasm

    15:1 occurrence rate (white:black)

    initially tumor is flat within choroid, with growth ruptures to give mushroom shape of solid tumor extending into vitreous (with overlying retina detached)

    smaller tumors (<10-mm diameter, 3-mm thickness)—relatively favorable prognosis

    treatment by enucleation controversial, most common site of metastasis—liver

    CT—highly accurate—well-defined hyperdense mass

    MR—moderate high SI on T_1, moderate low SI on T_2 (similar to retinoblastoma); imaging appearance due to paramagnetic melanin; retinal detachment better visualized than with CT

- uveal metastasis—often little thickening of uvea, one-third bilateral

- choroidal nevus—congenital, flat, most <2 mm, difficult to differentiate from melanoma
- choroidal hemangiomas—Sturge-Weber disease; enhancing ill-defined mass, may be concealed by retinal detachment
- retinal angiomas—von Hippel-Lindau disease; diagnosed by ophthalmoscopy
- senile macular degeneration—leading cause of legal blindness, arteriosclerosis of capillaries; thickening of Bruch's membrane, fluid in subretinal space, hemorrhage

---

224.892

Eyeball—retinal detachment

- posterior hyaloid detachment

    adults older than 50 years of age, macular degeneration

    fluid in this space shifts with position (that in vitreous does not)

    fluid in retrohyaloid space may be indistinguishable from that in subretinal space

- retinal detachment—sensory retina separated from retinal pigment epithelium (RPE)

    tear in sensory retina—cannot heal

    tear in RPE can heal (laser treatment for retinal detachment)

    causes—mass, fibroproliferative disease (diabetes), inflammatory process (*Toxocara*), Coats' disease (vascular anomaly of retina), trauma, senile macular degeneration

    imaging appearance—V-shaped with indentation at optic disk; ultrasound can be superior to CT and MR

    malignant melanoma, choroidal hemangioma—most common choroidal tumors to produce retinal detachment in adults

- choroidal detachment

    causes—surgery, trauma, inflammatory disease; can be due to fluid (serous detachment) or blood (hemorrhagic detachment)

    serous—cause is ocular hypotonia (with increased permeability of choroidal capillaries)—due to inflammation, perforation of eyeball, surgery, aggressive glaucoma therapy

    imaging appearance—smooth elevation of choroid from ciliary body posteriorly; serous—semilunar shape; hemorrhagic—low or high moundlike shape (lenticular); serous and hemorrhagic can be distinguished by both CT and MR

    may not be possible to differentiate subretinal and suprachoroidal fluid

Visual Pathways ....

229.11

Normal anatomy

- optic chiasm

axons from nasal half of retina cross to contralateral optic tract

axons from temporal half of retina do not cross

- visual field—right side (present on nasal half of right retina and temporal half of left retina) projects to left hemisphere (optic tract, geniculate nucleus [in thalamus], optic radiations, visual cortex), and vice versa
- lesion site/visual defect

  optic nerve/monocular blindness

  optic chiasm/bitemporal hemianopsia

  optic tract/contralateral homonymous hemianopsia

229.1211

CT technique

- IV contrast mandatory (unless trauma, foreign body, or history of contrast reaction)
- 5-mm axial sections from foramen magnum to orbit floor, 3-mm sections through orbit; 3-mm coronal sections

---

229.1214

MR technique

- technique of choice (vs. CT) except for trauma or foreign body
- IV contrast mandatory for neoplasia, inflammatory conditions, infection
- 3-mm axial T_1, T_2; 3-mm sagittal and coronal T_1; small FOV; fat suppression may be useful (for orbit)

229.22

Sarcoidosis

- clinical presentation—ophthalmic changes in up to 60%, lacrimal gland most frequently involved, cranial nerves commonly involved
- pathology—(noncaseating) granulomatous disease of unknown etiology, spreads along perivascular spaces

  two patterns of intracranial involvement:

  1. granulomatous leptomeningitis (with cranial nerve and hypothalamic involvement)
  2. nodules/parenchymal brain masses

- imaging appearance

  diffuse infiltration of leptomeninges (when intracranial), best seen with contrast enhancement

  enlargement and enhancement of cranial nerves

  homogeneously enhancing parenchymal nodules, with little edema, may be periventricular in location

  hydrocephalus due to obstruction of CSF outflow not uncommon

  enlargement of lacrimal gland (when intraorbital)

229.36

Neoplasm

.3611 Developmental origin—craniopharyngioma

- clinical presentation

    three age peaks: children (most common), young adults, fifth decade

    headache, visual disturbances, hypothalamic/pituitary dysfunction

- pathology—benign tumor arising from remnants of Rathke's pouch, well-encapsulated, cystic with solid portions

- imaging appearance

    location—suprasellar (may have intrasellar component)

    round, lobulated, irregularly marginated

    cystic components—85%, with variable attenuation and SI

    calcification—75% (by CT), conglomerate in nature

    marked contrast enhancement (solid components, rim)

.3619 Rathke's cleft cyst

- clinical presentation—small, asymptomatic
- pathology—benign cystic remnant of Rathke's pouch
- imaging appearance

    location—anterior in sella turcica or in suprasellar cistern

    cyst wall—thin, may enhance

    cyst contents—attenuation/SI similar to CSF

.363 Glial origin—optic glioma

- clinical presentation—first decade of life, 15% with neurofibromatosis, painless proptosis (when intraorbital), decreased vision
- pathology—grade I astrocytomas (juvenile pilocystic astrocytomas), slow-growing, do not metastasize
- imaging appearance

    smooth fusiform enlargement of optic nerve (may be kinking/buckling of nerve)

    unilateral or bilateral (latter with neurofibromatosis)

    frequent involvement of optic nerve, chiasm, and tract

    moderate contrast enhancement

.366 Perioptic meningioma

- clinical presentation—progressive monocular blindness, proptosis, diminished extraocular muscle motility
- pathology—pediatric lesions more aggressive than adult lesions
- imaging appearance

    eccentric mass along optic nerve or circumferential lesion (fusiform enlargement)

    intratumoral psammomatous (stippled) calcifications

bony hyperostosis

moderate-to-intense contrast enhancement

tram-track sign = enhancement of circumferential lesion

229.37

Intrasellar neoplasm—pituitary adenoma

- clinical presentation—bitemporal hemianopsia (large lesion with compression of chiasm), age 20–50, microadenomas with endocrine abnormalities, macroadenomas with mass effect (compression of chiasm or pituitary insufficiency)
- pathology

  benign, arise within pituitary gland, nonencapsulated, solid (may contain cystic, necrotic, or hemorrhagic areas)

  functional status—30% nonfunctional, 25% prolactin-secreting, 20% growth hormone-secreting, 10% adrenocorticotrophic hormone (ACTH)-secreting

- imaging appearance (high-field MR better than CT for detection/delineation)

  microadenomas—focal hypodense (CT)/hypointense (MR T_1) region; may deviate stalk, thin sellar floor, cause upward convexity of surface of gland; remain hypodense/hypointense on early post-contrast scans

  macroadenomas—enlarge sella, displace chiasm, mild uniform contrast enhancement

---

229.73

Ophthalmic artery aneurysm

- most common aneurysm to cause visual symptoms (due to impingement on visual pathway)
- clinical presentation

  subarachnoid hemorrhage (majority)

  visual symptoms (25%)

  > impaired visual acuity

  > visual field abnormalities

229.78

Infarct

- clinical presentation

  transient loss of vision in one eye (internal carotid artery [ICA] ischemia)

  contralateral homonymous hemianopsia (infarction in visual cortex, within occipital lobe)

229.871

Multiple sclerosis (MS)

- clinical presentation

    abnormal visual-evoked response—90%

    sudden onset of monocular blindness (optic neuritis)—20%

- imaging—use of fat suppression important for lesion demonstration in optic nerves by MR

Sinonasal Cavity...

23-26.11

Normal anatomy (sinonasal cavity)

- nasal cavity

    roof—cribriform plate

    floor—hard palate

    (olfactory mucosa—in upper nasal fossa, above level of superior turbinate)

    nasal septum—formed by ethmoid bone posteriorly, cartilage anteriorly, vomer posteroinferiorly

    lateral nasal wall (turbinate = concha, meatus = space lateral and beneath turbinate)

    > inferior turbinate—nasolacrimal duct opens into inferior meatus

    > middle turbinate—nasofrontal duct (draining frontal sinus) opens into middle meatus in 50%, into ethmoids in 50% (which then drain into middle meatus); hiatus semilunaris—a slit in middle meatus into which maxillary sinus drains (antral ostium is high on medial sinus wall)

    > superior turbinate—posterior ethmoids drain into superior meatus

    > supreme turbinate (seen in only 60% of patients)

    "nasal cycle"—alternation of nasal function with time, from left to right side

    vascular supply—from both external and internal carotid arteries; for nasal lining, supply from sphenopalatine artery is most important

- paranasal sinuses

    frontal sinus—each sinus is usually a single cavity, typically asymmetric in size, larger sinus can cross midline, septum (dividing the two sinuses) usually midline at base

    ethmoid sinuses—3 to 18 cells (adult); divided into anterior, middle, and posterior ethmoid air-cell groups

    sphenoid sinus—degree of pneumatization varies widely; in 60% extends below sella; if >1–2 mm bone between sinus and anterior sella wall, transphenoidal hypophysectomy is not possible (< 1% of population); septum is midline anteriorly, but can deviate to one side posteriorly; in about ½, lateral recesses extend into greater sphenoid wing

maxillary sinus—tend to develop symmetrically, but unilateral and bilateral hypoplasia do occur

---

23–26.11

Imaging technique and related anatomy (sinonasal cavity)

.11   plain film (technique)

- horizontal beam, 5° off-lateral view

    allows identification of air-fluid levels

    5° rotation—so posterior walls of maxillary antra are not superimposed (and can be examined individually)

- Caldwell view (a frontal projection)

    patient faces cassette

    orbitomeatal line is perpendicular to cassette

    beam angled 15° caudally as it enters posteriorly—petrous pyramids project over lower orbits

    best frontal projection to examine frontal and ethmoid sinuses

    superior orbital fissure and foramen rotundum (latter seen superiorly and medially in antrum) well-depicted

- Waters view (a frontal projection)

    patient faces cassette

    orbitomeatal line is angled 37° relative to cassette

    beam is perpendicular to cassette—petrous pyramids project just below floor of sinuses

    best frontal projection to examine maxillary sinuses

- base (submentovertex) view

    infraorbitomeatal line (line from infraorbital margin to external auditory meatus) parallel to cassette

    used for examination of sphenoid and ethmoid sinuses

- oblique (Rhese) view

    patient faces cassette (film centered on orbit)

    canthomeatal line perpendicular to film

    head rotated 53°

    beam angled 15° caudally as it enters posteriorly

    best projection for study of posterior ethmoid air cells

- nasal bone views—lateral and axial

plain film (interpretation)

- only that portion of sinus wall parallel to beam is depicted (role for multiple plain film views and/or cross-sectional imaging)
- small sinus (hypoplastic)—will appear "clouded," even if normal, thus difficult to evaluate
- loss of scalloped margins (frontal and maxillary sinuses)—suggests expansile process
- mucoperiosteal line (normal structure)—thin (1 mm) dense rim, outlining sinus, separating sinus from adjacent bone—lost in active infection

- oblique orbital lines (linea innominata)—seen in Waters and Caldwell views, correspond to anterior part of medial temporal fossa
- consistently underestimates extent of soft tissue disease and bone erosion (vs. cross-sectional imaging)

.12 Cross-sectional imaging

- CT

    both soft tissue and bone windows are important, latter also most accurate for assessment of air-soft tissue interfaces

    preferred scan plane (axial)—parallel to inferior orbitomeatal line

    additional coronal scans mandated when visualization of floor of anterior cranial fossa, orbital floor, and hard palate necessary for surgery

    postcontrast studies advocated for improved differentiation of normal tissue and pathology

- MR

    superior soft tissue differentiation vs. CT

    inferior depiction of fine bony change

23-26.2

Inflammation (sinonasal cavity)

- etiology

    acute bacterial sinusitis

    preceding viral infection ("common cold")

    turbinate swelling may cause sinus ostium obstruction, leading to acute bacterial sinusitis

    dental infection or tooth extraction

- clinical presentation/pathology

    acute bacterial sinusitis

    pain (over affected sinus)

    mucopurulent discharge

    asymmetric involvement—disease often unilateral or isolated to single sinus

    (pediatric patient—sinus opacification and mucosal thickening of questionable value in diagnosis)

    chronic sinusitis

    repeated or persistent infection, can be atrophy or hypertrophy of mucosa, bony sinus walls become thick and sclerotic

    allergic sinusitis

    symmetrical involvement

    nasal polyposis (differentiating point from bacterial sinusitis)

    profuse secretions with resultant obstruction can lead to bacterial sinusitis

- imaging appearance

    sinus mucosa

normal—so thin as not to be seen on plain films, CT, or MR

thickened—causes = fibrosis, inflammation (allergy), infection, and tumor

plain film—clouding of sinus (seen early), uniform thickening (with disease progression)

disease of ethmoids and sphenoid sinus—poorly depicted

CT

no enhancement of thickened mucosa—usually edema (allergy) or fibrosis

thin zone of surface enhancement with submucosal edema—active infection

MR

low SI on T_1, high SI on T_2—inflammation

high T_2 SI differentiates this from tumor (intermediate T_2 SI) and fibrosis (low T_2 SI)

- air-fluid level

most common location = maxillary sinuses

etiology

most common = acute bacterial sinusitis

other causes

sinus lavage

trauma

mucosal tear with blood

placement of nasotracheal or nasogastric tube, combined with bed rest

barotrauma (aviators, divers)

complications

meningitis, brain infection—can occur in anterior cranial fossa within 48 hours of recognition of frontal sinusitis, due to rich venous network

- cysts, polyps—most common local complication of inflammation; cannot be distinguished (cyst vs. intrasinus polyp) by imaging; when large, begin to resemble on imaging an air-fluid level (close attention demanded to direction of gravity and inspection of border, which should be slightly convex)

mucous retention cyst—most common of all cysts and polyps

caused by obstruction of seromucinous gland

maxillary sinus—most common location

incidental finding

polyp—local upheaval of mucosa (extracellular water accumulation)

etiologies—inflammatory, allergic

allergic—usually multiple polyps

most common expansile lesion of nasal cavity

when chronic, with progression of size, can cause extensive deformation and bone destruction when form conglomerate mass—difficult to differentiate from tumor

if in ethmoids, widening of complex without destruction of delicate septae (by CT) signifies benign disease

if separated from adjacent bone by mucoid material (by CT)—also signifies benign disease (vs. tumor, which abuts bone or destroys bone)

imaging

CT—mucoid attenuation (with occasional mucosal enhancement along surface)

MR—low T_1 SI, high T_2 SI

when chronic, may have mixed SI on all sequences

very proteinaceous collections may manifest signal void

(mycetoma—low SI on all sequences)

antrochoanal polyp

5% of all polyps

due to expansion of polyp, with prolapse through sinus ostium

- fungal disease

etiology—most common = aspergillosis, mucormycosis, candidiasis

aspergillosis

usually involves maxillary sinus, with formation of aspergilloma (mat of tangled hyphae)

mucormycosis

occurs in poorly controlled diabetes and in other chronic disease states

black, necrotic tissue

treatment with amphotericin B

candidiasis

severe infections—occur in immunocompromised patients

imaging appearance

in early stages, nonspecific findings

involvement of soft tissues of cheek or face is suggestive of fungal disease

- granulomatous disease

etiology

actinomycosis—usually spreads to sinus from apical (tooth) disease/abscess

tuberculosis—involvement of sinuses is usually secondary to pulmonary disease

syphilis

South American blastomycosis

leprosy

Wegener's granulomatosis—a necrotizing vasculitis

idiopathic (lethal) midline granuloma—a chronic necrotizing inflammation of nose, sinuses, midface, and upper airways

cocaine abuse—causes necrotizing vasculitis, with subsequent granuloma, of nasal septum (long-term exposure produces septal erosion)

imaging appearance—ranges from nonspecific inflammation to soft tissue mass, paranasal sinuses usually involved after nasal fossa

- mucoceles—most common expansile lesion involving a paranasal sinus

    etiology/pathology

    cuboidal epithelium surrounding mucoid secretions

    obstruction of sinus ostium (or compartment in a septated sinus)

    incidence—frontal > ethmoid > maxillary > sphenoid

    imaging appearance

    plain film—radiodensity equal or slightly less than normal sinus (due to bone erosion); significant off-midline posterior extension (frontal sinus lesion) can be missed on lateral plain film

    preoperative cross-sectional imaging mandated

    CT—expanded sinus (remodeled walls), mucoid attenuation

    MR—low T_1 SI (if present for long time, SI on T_1 may be high—due to protein content and resorption of water), high T_2 SI

- cholesteatoma

    etiology/pathology

    cystic mass with wall of stratified squamous epithelium and keratin centrally

    origin—congenital rest or post-traumatic implant

    imaging appearance

    plain film—lucent, scalloped margins, thin white border

    CT—expansile, mucoid attenuation

    MR—high T_1 SI, intermediate T_2 SI (fat)

- complications (from paranasal sinusitis)

    orbital/preseptal inflammation (including cavernous sinus thrombosis)

    orbital infection—most often from ethmoid involvement

    intracranial complications—meningitis, abscess

    most often from frontal involvement

    osteomyelitis (in patients with chronic disease)

22-26.41

Fracture (sinonasal cavity)

- complications

    osteomyelitis (0.5%)

    sinusitis (8%)

- imaging—CT (axial and coronal)

22.41

Orbital fracture

- blow-out: object too large to enter orbit
    - orbit content ruptures into maxillary sinus
    - antral opacification
    - globe usually undamaged
    - diplopia—edema/hemorrhage or entrapment of muscles
    - often accompanied by medial wall fracture—inferred by orbital emphysema
- blow-in: (rare) orbital floor fracture fragments herniate into orbit

231.41

Frontal sinus fracture

- majority limited to anterior table

234.41

Sphenoid sinus fracture

- rare, associated with severe trauma and basilar skull fractures

241.41

Maxillary fracture

- alveolar—most common

242.41

Zygomatic (trimalar) fracture

- along zygomaticofrontal suture, inferior orbital fissure, anterior and posterior maxillary walls, zygomaticotemporal suture

261.41

Nasal fractures

- most common fracture of face
- involve distal third of nasal bone (most commonly)
- injury to lateral cartilaginous walls not seen by x-ray

268.41

Midface fracture

- LeFort I
    - blow over upper lip

detachment of upper jaw with tooth-bearing segments and caudal maxillary sinuses

- LeFort II

  blow over central face

  fracture through nose root, lacrimal bones, medial orbit walls, orbit floor, zygomaticomaxillary suture, anterior maxilla wall, lower pterygoid plates

  zygomatic bones remain attached to skull base

- LeFort III

  separation of facial skeleton from skull base

22-26.45

Postoperative (sinonasal cavity)

- importance of baseline studies
- CT is exam of choice

  IV contrast used to differentiate inflammation, tumor, and scar

---

231.45

Frontal sinus surgery

- acute infection

  trephination—incision and drainage

- chronic infection—nonobliterative surgery—Lynch, Killian's, and Ridell's procedures
- chronic infection—obliterative osteoplastic flap procedure

  less cosmetically deforming (vs. nonobliterative surgery)

  CT can visualize bone flap (anterior sinus wall)

  sinus mucosa removed, sinus obliterated with fat

232.45

Ethmoid sinus surgery

- three approaches, all which remove ethmoid septae

  external

  absent anterior lamina papyracea

  internal (intranasal)

  absent medial ethmoid wall, middle turbinate

  transmaxillary

  Caldwell-Luc defect, absent medial upper antral wall

233.45

Maxillary sinus surgery

- endoscopic technique
- intranasal antrostomy

- Caldwell-Luc procedure—bony defect in lower anterior sinus wall; membrane can form obstructing lateral maxillary sinus, leading to mucocele
- Krönlein operation—lateral orbitotomy; for thyroid ophthalmopathy

---

234.45

Sphenoid sinus surgery

- opens anterior wall of sinus, which then communicates with nasopharynx
- intranasal, transmaxillary, transseptal, transethmoidal approaches
- risk of carotid artery damage (aneurysm, carotid-cavernous fistula)

239.45

Surgery for malignancy

- partial maxillectomy—normal mucosa lines the defect
- total maxillectomy (may include orbital exenteration)—split thickness graft lines the defect
- nasoethmoid surgery—lateral rhinotomy provides access to nasal cavity, maxillary, ethmoid, and sphenoid sinuses; medial antral wall, ethmoid cells, inferior and middle turbinates removed
- craniofacial resection—frontal craniotomy, resection of middle part of floor of anterior cranial fossa, lateral rhinotomy

---

23-26.3

Neoplasm (and neoplastic-like disease)—sinonasal cavity

- frequently present with advanced stage
- often accompanied by chronic inflammatory disease (and thus overlooked)

     CT with contrast—important for differentiation

     MR (T_2)—more valuable than enhanced CT for differentiation

          most inflammatory change is high SI (T_2), while most sinonasal tumors are highly cellular with intermediate SI (T_2)

- clinical symptoms—visual symptoms, nasal stuffiness, epistaxis, mass
- surgical/treatment approach—altered by extension into anterior/middle cranial fossae, pterygopalatine fossa, orbit, or palate
- bone involvement

     aggressive bone destruction—squamous cell carcinoma most likely, also metastases

     bone remodeling—sarcoma, mucocele, polyps, inverted papilloma, minor salivary gland tumors, lymphoma, esthesioneuroblastoma, hemangiopericytoma

- nodal metastasis—grave prognostic sign

.312 Osteoma

- benign proliferation of bone, principally occurs in frontal sinus (other locations—ethmoid > maxillary > sphenoid), bone density varies (compact vs. cancellous vs. fibrous types), incidental finding on plain film, almost all remain confined to sinus, multiple lesions (skull, mandible)—think Gardner's syndrome

.322 Osteogenic sarcoma (osteosarcoma)

- second most common malignant tumor of skeleton after multiple myeloma
- of head and neck lesions, most in mandible and maxilla
- vary from lytic to blastic in appearance
- classic "sunburst" periosteal bone reaction (rapid tumor growth)

.321 Cartilaginous origin tumors (chondroma, chondrosarcoma)

- rare in sinonasal cavity, but usually malignant (vs. larynx)

.34 Lymphoma

- approximately 5% occur in sinonasal cavity
- radiocurable
- bulky lesions
- moderate contrast enhancement (CT)

.3451 Extramedullary plasmacytoma

- rare soft tissue tumor (made up of plasma cells), uncommon in sinonasal cavity; homogenous, enhance, remodel bone, polypoid in shape

.3452 Plasma cell dyscrasias

- multiple myeloma—most common of this group
    proliferation of tumor cells in red marrow, destroys bone (lytic lesions)
    soft tissue involvement can occur

.362 Hemangioma

- present with epistaxis (severe) or nasal obstruction, usually small and in nasal cavity, simple excision is curative

.364 Neurogenic tumors

- schwannoma (= neuroma = neurinoma = neurilemoma = perineural fibroblastoma)
    benign, encapsulated, slowly growing, nerve sheath tumor
    common in head and neck, uncommon in sinonasal cavity
    two major histologic types—Antoni type A (compact cells) and type B (loose myxoid stroma)
    remodel bone
    nerve may be spared at surgery
- neurofibroma
    benign, well-circumscribed, nonencapsulated
    may be solitary or multiple with or without neurofibromatosis

malignant degeneration seen in 10%

CT—variable appearance due to cystic regions, fatty replacement, and enhancement of solid portion

remodel bone

nerve is integral part of tumor

.3661 Meningioma—less than 1% occur outside brain or spine

.369 Other benign soft tissue neoplasms

- papilloma—*not* associated with allergy, infection, or smoking

    most common types:

    1. fungiform—not premalignant
    2. inverted

        arise from lateral nasal wall, near middle turbinate, extend secondarily into sinuses (maxillary, ethmoid)

        symptoms—nasal obstruction, epistaxis, anosmia

        local surgery—high recurrence rate

        associated malignancy—>10%

- angiofibroma ("nasopharyngeal" or "juvenile" angiofibroma)

    highly vascular, nonencapsulated, polypoid, histologically benign, locally aggressive, enhancing lesion (CT/MR)

    clinical presentation

        males

        age 10–18 years

        nasal obstruction, epistaxis

    origin—nasopharynx near pterygopalatine and sphenopalatine fossa

    imaging—majority demonstrate

        widening of pterygopalatine fossa, with anterior bowing of posterior antral wall

        involvement of sphenoid sinus

        angiography—major feeders = internal maxillary and ascending pharyngeal arteries (on dominant side)

    intracranial extent in 5–20%

- angiomatous polyp—fibrous vascular nasal (*not* nasopharyngeal) polyp resulting from trauma

.37 Malignant soft tissue neoplasms

- squamous cell carcinoma

    distribution (incidence)—maxillary sinus > nasal cavity > ethmoid sinus

    presentation—> age 40, twice as common in men as women

    imaging—bone destruction seen in majority

- adenoid cystic carcinoma—perineural spread characteristic, clean surgical margins have little prognostic significance, high recurrence rate (may recur late), most common of minor salivary gland tumors in sinonasal cavity

- other glandular tumors—after adenoid cystic carcinoma, in incidence adenocarcinoma > mucoepidermoid carcinoma > benign mixed tumors (pleomorphic adenoma)
- olfactory neuroblastoma (esthesioneuroblastoma)

  broad age range

  polypoid, may bleed profusely

  tumor may be present intracranially (microscopically) despite intact cribriform plate

  CT—homogeneous, enhancing, remodel bone

.371 Malignant melanoma

- most arise from nasal septum
- age 50–70 years
- treatment—wide surgical excision
- > 50% present with metastases within 1 year
- remodel bone
- CT/MR—prominent enhancement

.374 Sarcoma

- rhabdomyosarcoma—primarily pediatric in nature, tumor of striated muscle, embryonal type arises in first decade of life
- fibrosarcoma—most arise in lower extremities and trunk

.652 Thalassemia

- thickened calvarium, hair-on-end appearance, in face may have delayed sinus pneumatization and expansion of maxilla (both due to marrow expansion)

.84 Paget's disease

- occurs in patients over age 50 years
- calvarium involved in about half (may involve in addition maxilla and mandible)

  neurologic abnormalities due to reduced size of cranial cavity

.85 Fibrous dysplasia

- medullary bone replaced by poorly organized, fibro-osseous tissue
- bone expansion can compromise sinuses, orbits, neurovascular canals

Mandible ....

243.11

Mandible—normal anatomy

- body
- ascending ramus; masseter inserts on outer cortex, medial pterygoid on inner cortex
- coronoid process; temporalis muscle inserts anteriorly

- condyle—head and neck; lateral pterygoid muscle inserts anteriorly on neck
- tooth socket (alveolus) surrounded by cancellous bone; alveolus lined by dense cortical bone = cribriform plate = lamina dura; between lamina dura and tooth = periodontal ligament = lucent zone
- deciduous teeth (20 total)—two incisors, one canine, two molars in each quadrant
- permanent teeth (32 total)—two incisors, one canine, two premolars, three molars in each quadrant

243.11

Mandible—plain film

- posteroanterior view
- lateral oblique view—most common, useful projection
- lateral view
- panoramic view—survey of entire mandible and maxilla
- intraoral films—nonscreen high-speed film; three projections— periapical (details anatomy of tooth apex and adjacent bone), bitewing, occlusal

243.1211

Mandible—CT

- axial and coronal planes
- assessment of tumors within and adjacent to bone

243.1214

Mandible—MR

- axial and coronal planes
- assessment of extraosseous lesion extent
- obliteration of marrow high SI on T_1 implies tumor invasion

243.381

Dental cyst—odontogenic (from tooth derivatives) vs. nonodontogenic

- odontogenic

    periodontal—includes periapical (radicular) and lateral cysts

    radicular—most common odontogenic cyst, occurs with untreated caries

    dentigerous (follicular)—second most common odontogenic cyst, occurs with crown of unerupted tooth; osteolysis

    odontogenic keratocyst—body/ramus of mandible, high recurrence rate, occurs with impacted tooth

    basal cell nevus syndrome—at least two of following: multiple cysts of jaw, multiple basal cell carcinomas, ectopic calcifications (falx, dura), skeletal abnormalities

- nonodontogenic

    fissural: (1) incisive canal = nasopalatine duct cyst—fourth to sixth decades, midline, round or oval; (2) globulomaxillary—between lateral incisor and canine, pear shaped

    solitary (simple, or hemorrhagic)—young patients, from injury without fracture

    Stafne bone cyst (static bone cavity)—angle of mandible, asymptomatic, open to lingual surface

---

243.382

Cementoblastoma, cementoma

- periapical cemental dysplasia—well-defined radiolucency at tooth apex which transforms with time into radiopaque mass
- benign cementoblastoma—younger than 25 years of age, dense radiopaque central tumor attached to tooth root

---

243.384

Odontoma

- benign, contains tissue components of teeth (enamel, dentin, cementum, pulp)—arranged in disorderly pattern, frequently associated with unerupted teeth, second and third decades

---

243.385

Ameloblastoma (adamantinoma)

- benign, odontogenic; third and fourth decades; 80% in mandible; slow-growing, painless; radiolucent, multi- or unilocular; oval with distinct borders, can cause extensive destruction, tendency to break through cortex with formation of soft tissue mass

---

243.389

Other

- odontogenic myxoma—second, third decades, painless, slow-growing, can cause marked expansion and destruction, radiolucent lesion septated by bony trabeculae
- benign nonodontogenic tumors

    exostoses—localized outgrowth of bone; three types: torus mandibularis (lingual surface of mandible), torus palatinus (midline —hard palate), multiple exostoses

    osteoma—benign neoplasm, compact or cancellous bone, well-circumscribed sclerotic bony mass; Gardner's syndrome—multiple osteomas and polyposis of colon

    giant cell granuloma—radiolucent, multilocular, honeycombed appearance

    eosinophilic granuloma—males, third decade, punched-out area of osteolysis

- fibro-osseous lesions

    fibrous dysplasia—more common in maxilla than mandible, first three decades of life, bony expansion, homogenous, may be radiopaque

- malignant tumors

    carcinoma—origin in oral cavity or maxillary sinus, with secondary invasion

    metastasis—soft tissue and bony swelling, teeth loss

    osteogenic sarcoma—most osteoblastic

    multiple myeloma—punched-out, ovoid radiolucencies

Temporomandibular Joints ....

244.11

Temporomandibular joint (TMJ)—normal anatomy

- osseous components

    mandibular condyle

    glenoid fossa

    articular tubercle

- TMJ disc

    biconcave

    thick periphery, thin center

    sagittal plane—disk appears biconcave

    coronal plane—disk appears crescent-shaped

    anterior and posterior parts of disk = anterior and posterior bands

    normal position—posterior band located at 12:00 over condyle

    posterior disk attachment (= bilaminar zone)—is to temporal bone and condyle

    upper (predominantly for translation) and lower (predominantly for rotation) joint compartments

    during all motion—central thin portion of disk remains between condyle and articular tubercle

244.42

Internal derangement (TMJ)

- typically = disk displacement

    most often—anterior or anteromedial

- types of disk displacement

    anterior

    anteromedial rotational

    anterolateral rotational

    medial sideways

    lateral sideways

- displacement can occur with or without reduction; reduction = disk reverts to normal position on opening

- disk displacement with reduction—"click" on opening = reduction
- disk displacement without reduction—disk remains displaced regardless of jaw position; limited jaw opening and deviation to affected side only in early disease stage
- disk deformation—late disease stages, disk becomes biconvex; communication between upper and lower joint spaces also occurs—perforation usually in posterior disk attachment; osseous changes—flattening of condyle, osteophytes

---

244.11

TMJ—plain film

- transcranial projection (lateral)—lateral part of joint well-depicted
- anteroposterior projection—transmaxillary or transorbital

244.1218

TMJ—tomography

- for osseous anatomy
- large radiation dose to lens
- largely replaced by CT

244.122

TMJ—arthrography

- single-contrast lower-compartment arthrography—most common arthrographic technique at present
- double contrast—air and iodine, both joint compartments, technically more difficult; requires tomography
- indications

    assess position and function of disk—in patient with pain

    assess position of mandible that achieves disk reduction—for protrusive splint therapy
- technique—single contrast

    lower joint space punctured (at superoposterior aspect of condyle) with 23-gauge needle, 0.2–0.5 ml non-ionic contrast injected

    spot films in open and closed mouth positions, videotaping of opening and closing
- technique—double contrast

    lower joint entered as in single-joint technique with 0.8 mm angiocath, upper joint entered along posterior slope of tubercle with 0.8 mm angiocath; 0.2–0.5 ml contrast for each joint space

    videofluoroscopy as with single joint technique

    aspirate contrast, inject air, obtain tomograms in open and closed positions
- findings

    enlargement of anterior recess of lower joint compartment in disk displacement extensive disk deformity (late disease)

perforation (late disease)—directly visualized on double-contrast study or by flow to upper joint in single-contrast study

loose bodies—synovial chondromatosis, osteochondritis dessicans, osteoarthrosis

244.1211

TMJ—CT

- technique—direct sagittal preferred over axial with reconstructions; coronal reconstructions; closed and open mouth views
- best means of examining osseous joint structures
- normal appearance—disk difficult to visualize
- anterior displacement—disk is high attenuation mass anterior to condyle within pterygoid fat pad; high incidence of false negative studies

244.1214

TMJ—MR

- technique

    dual surface coils (both joints)

    closed and open mouth views in sagittal and coronal planes— relative to the joint itself—(T_1 or proton density); T_2-weighting for tissue edema or joint fluid

- normal appearance—disk has low SI; posterior disk distinguished from posterior disk attachment by fat component of latter
- MR preferred over arthrography for evaluation of TMJ (unless joint dynamics are primary concern)
- abnormal findings

    disk displacement

    late stage degenerative bony and soft tissue changes

    abnormal position of disk during incremental opening/closing (assessed with rapid GRE scans)

    avascular necrosis of mandibular condyle—low SI on T_1 of marrow

- postoperative—MR is modality of choice for evaluation of possible surgical complications

    disk correctly repositioned?

    evaluation of granulation tissue and bony deformities with disk implant

Nasopharynx, Oral Cavity, Oropharynx..................

26.11

Pharynx and oral cavity—embryology

- pharyngeal arches—first to sixth, give rise to bone, muscles, nerves, thyroid gland

- pharyngeal pouches—first to fifth, give rise to parenchymal organs—including parathyroids, thymus gland, some thyroid cells
- pharyngeal clefts—first to fourth, give rise to ectodermal structures including external auditory meatus
- tongue—anterior two thirds (derived from first pharyngeal arch) innervated by mandibular segment of trigeminal nerve, posterior one third (derived from second–fourth pharyngeal arches) by glossopharyngeal nerve

---

263.11

Nasopharynx—normal anatomy

- borders of the nasopharynx

    roof—sphenoid sinus and upper clivus

    posterior margin—lower clivus and upper cervical spine

    anterior margin—nasal cavity

    lateral walls—pterygoid plates (anteriorly), fascia and muscle of airway (posteriorly)

    floor—separated from oropharynx by soft palate

- levator, tensor veli palatini muscles—arise from skull base, attach to soft palate, elevate and tense the palate
- pharyngobasilar fascia—holds airway patent; surrounds mucosa, superior constrictor, levator palatini muscles; divides superficial mucosal space from deep fascial spaces
- superficial (mucosal) space

    contains—mucosa, adenoidal tissue (in superior recesses), superior and middle constrictor muscles, torus tubarius, levator palatini muscle; minor salivary glands abundant

    mucosa and adenoidal tissue—intermediate SI on T_1, high SI on T_2

    eustachian tubes end in torus tubarius (a lateral cartilaginous enlargement)

    lateral pharyngeal recess of Rosenmueller—formed by mucosal reflection over longus colli and capitis muscles (flexors of cervical spine)—site of origin for 50% of squamous cell carcinoma of nasopharynx

    levator palatini muscle—just lateral to torus, separated by fat plane from longus muscles

    tensor palatini muscle—lateral to pharyngobasilar fascia and levator muscle, surrounded by fat

- deep musculofascial spaces (nasopharynx and oropharynx)

    parapharyngeal space

        triangular fat-filled space deep to pharyngobasilar fascia

        in direct continuity with basisphenoid and inferior petrous apex, submandibular and parotid glands

        contains CN V_3, pharyngeal artery and vein branches

        displacement: lateral implies lesion of superficial or mucosal origin, medial by masses in deep parotid or masticator space, anterior by masses in carotid space

carotid space

> from skull base to aortic arch
>
> enclosed by carotid sheath
>
> contains internal carotid artery, internal jugular vein (right greater than left in size in 80% of patients), CN IX-XII, sympathetic plexus, lateral retropharyngeal lymph nodes

masticator space

> contains muscles of mastication (lateral and medial pterygoids, temporalis, masseter—all innervated by CN V_3), ramus and posterior body of mandible, pterygoid venous plexus
>
> route for infection and tumor to skull base

prevertebral space—between deep layer of cervical fascia and vertebral bodies, extends from skull base to coccyx, contains vertebral column and prevertebral muscles

parotid space

retropharyngeal space—potential space between prevertebral muscles and pharyngeal constrictor muscles

---

262.11

Oral cavity and oropharynx—normal anatomy

- oral cavity—anterior two thirds of tongue, buccal mucosa, floor of mouth
- oropharynx—posterior one third of tongue (base), palatine tonsils, lymphoid tissue at base of tongue, soft palate, oropharyngeal mucosa, constrictor muscles
- T_1—best contrast for muscle vs. fat, T_2—best contrast for muscle vs. lymphoid tissue
- floor of mouth—combination of following muscles: mylohyoid (sling-shaped) and anterior belly of digastric and geniohyoid and intrinsic muscles of tongue (genioglossal, styloglossal, hyoglossal)—all innervated by CN XII

26.1211

Pharynx, oral cavity—CT

- preferred for study of oral cavity (less motion vs. MR)
- naso- and oropharynx—studied with suspended respiration
- IV contrast—for lesion margins, vascularity, normal vessel enhancement

---

26.1214

Pharynx, oral cavity—MR

- imaging modality of choice for study of nasopharynx
- scans of naso- and oropharynx with head coil, scans of neck with neck coil (using both anterior and posterior components)
- axial scans (T_1 and T_2), supplemented with coronal T_1 images

262.2

Oral Cavity, Oropharynx—inflammation

- most inflammatory disease—due to infections of teeth, mandible, salivary glands (obstructive calculus), or tonsils
- Ludwig's angina—extensive infection of floor of mouth
- acute tonsillitis (self-limited disease of the young), tonsillar abscess

262.36

Oral Cavity, Oropharynx—benign lesions

- lingual thyroid—dorsal posterior one third of tongue most common site of ectopic thyroid
- hemangioma—children, tongue base
- benign masseteric hypertrophy—half are bilateral
- neurogenic tumors
    - schwannoma, neurofibroma
    - granular cell tumors
    - minor salivary gland tumors (50% malignant)

262.37

Oral Cavity, Oropharynx—malignant tumors

- types
    - > 90% squamous cell carcinoma—anterior more benign, posterior more malignant; association with alcohol, tobacco use; many infiltrate deeply
    - 5% lymphoma (non-Hodgkins)—indistinguishable from squamous cell carcinoma on imaging
    - minor salivary gland carcinomas
- routes of spread (squamous cell carcinoma)—submucosally and along deep musculofascial planes
- characteristics by location
    - tongue
        - easy spread along intrinsic muscles
        - rich lymphatics—high incidence of bilateral lymph node involvement
        - important to assess spread across midline, as hemiglossectomy is surgical option
    - floor of mouth—majority squamous, bilateral lymph node involvement common
    - palate
        - majority squamous
        - minor salivary gland carcinomas—highest incidence in posterior soft palate
        - 60% with lymphatic spread at time of diagnosis

MR superior to CT; coronal and sagittal T_1s (abundant normal fat in palate)

tonsil

> most common location for carcinoma in oropharynx and oral cavity
>
> elderly men with cigarette, alcohol history
>
> highly malignant, tendency for early metastases, 75% with nodal metastases at presentation, bilateral spread common

base of tongue

> usually delayed diagnosis
>
> poor prognosis
>
> bilateral adenopathy in 30%
>
> as with oral-tongue lesions, high SI on T_2

pharyngeal walls—aggressive squamous cell carcinoma with tendency to bilateral nodal metastases; thickening of pharyngeal wall over several cm characteristic

---

263.2

Nasopharynx—inflammation

- masticator space infection—results from osteomyelitis of mandible (due to dental infection); surrounding cellulitis
- malignant otitis externa—elderly diabetics (*Pseudomonas aeruginosa*); nasopharyngeal mass, skull-base osteomyelitis, obliteration of external auditory canal by soft tissue
- retropharyngeal abscess—from tonsillar infection in children (IV contrast—differentiation of frank abscess from cellulitis)
- parapharyngeal space abscess—from tonsillar infection or perforation of pharynx, mycotic aneurysm of carotid artery can result if not drained

---

263.36–7

Nasopharynx—soft tissue masses (benign and malignant)

- benign, "incidental"

  adenoidal hypertrophy—children, young adults

  Tornwaldt's cyst—4% at autopsy, midline cyst 1–5 mm diameter, high SI on T_1 and T_2 (proteinaceous fluid)

- mucosal space masses

  squamous cell carcinoma

  > 80% of superficial epithelial carcinomas of nasopharynx
  >
  > prevalent in Asia
  >
  > lateral pharyngeal recess—most common site of origin
  >
  > can grow inferiorly, superiorly (skull-base erosion), anteriorly, posteriorly; lateral extension—most common
  >
  > 80% with nodal involvement on presentation; metastatic spread suspected in adults when retropharyngeal nodes > 5 mm diameter (or with necrotic node—seen on T_2 or with IV contrast)

               ipsilateral mastoid opacification, otitis media common

               perineural tumor spread

               therapy—radiation—result is fibrosis with low SI on T_1 and T_2

          lymphoma (non-Hodgkins)—rarely involves only nasopharynx

          rhabdomyosarcoma—30% involve head and neck; of these—most common in orbit or nasopharynx; children < 6 years of age; invasion of skull base, local recurrence, distant metastases all common

- deep compartment masses

          carotid space masses (benign)

               paraganglioma (arise from amine precursor uptake, decarboxylase [APUD] cells—secrete norepinephrine, epinephrine, serotonin)

                    characteristic symptoms—hypertension, blushing, tachycardia

                    common sites—carotid bifurcation, jugular bulb, middle ear (tympanicum), vagus nerve (nodose ganglion)

                    5% multiple; 20% family history

                    irregular and permeative bone destruction

                    CT, MR—intense enhancement

                    MR—heterogeneous with high and low SI foci on T_2

               schwannoma—usually single, may cause pain and neuropathy; smooth scalloping of adjacent bone; necrosis or cystic change in large lesions characteristic; intense enhancement on MR

               neurofibroma—10% of patients have neurofibromatosis

               meningioma (rare, can extend to carotid space via jugular fossa)

- parapharyngeal space masses—true primary tumors in this space are rare

          lipoma

          minor salivary gland tumor

Salivary Glands ....

264.11

Salivary glands—normal anatomy

- major salivary glands—parotid, submandibular, sublingual

2641.11

Parotid gland

- smaller, deep portion—between mandibular ramus, sternocleidomastoid muscle, and posterior belly of digastric muscle
- no true superficial and deep lobes—convention uses facial nerve to artifically divide these regions
- main parotid duct—Stensen's—opens opposite second upper molar, 6 cm long
- pure serous gland

2642.11

Submandibular gland

- main duct—Wharton's—opens onto anterior floor of mouth on sublingual papilla, 5 cm long
- mixed serous and mucous gland

2643.11

Minor salivary glands

- concentrated in buccal, labial, lingual, palatal regions
- predominantly mucous glands

264.11

Salivary glands—plain films

- used to detect:
    radiopaque sialolithiasis
    dystrophic calcifications
    mandibular bone disease

264.121

Salivary glands—CT/MR

- exam of choice for mass lesions—can evaluate:
    presence of mass
    location, position relative to facial nerve
    margin of mass—smooth or infiltrating
    confined to gland or extension into neck
    necrotic, cystic, solid
    determine if one mass vs. bilateral disease (clinically silent)
- external carotid artery, posterior facial vein—posterior to ramus of mandible
- mass with focal calcifications on CT—benign mixed tumor
- highly cellular tumors (high-grade)—intermediate SI on MR vs. less cellular (benign, low-grade)—high SI on T_2
- malignant tumors—hard, fixed on palpation, often facial nerve paralysis
- both CT and MR highly sensitive for detecting salivary gland masses

264.1222

Sialography

- parotid or submandibular glands
- used for diseases with distinctive ductal findings—sialadenitis, autoimmune disease, sialosis

- contraindicated in infection
- indications

    detect sialoliths, foreign bodies

    evaluate irreversible ductal damage (infection)

    disease differentiation

    evaluate fistulas, strictures, ductal anatomy

    dilating procedure for stenosis

- use water-soluble agents—Sinografin

    evacuation film should show complete, rapid ductal emptying

---

264.2

Salivary glands—inflammation

- viral and bacterial disease—most common salivary gland abnormality
- parotid gland most commonly involved
- mumps—most common viral parotitis; bilateral (two-thirds)
- bacterial infection—two-thirds are postoperative (but not following oral surgery) due to poor oral hygiene, debilitation, dehydration; treatment —antibiotics
- sialodochitis—inflammation of main salivary duct
- CT

    bacterial infection—enlarged gland, increased attenuation; scattered contrast collections on sialogram consistent with abscesses

    sialodochitis—enlarged Stensen's duct, enhancing walls

- sialolithiasis

    salivary gland stones—80% submandibular, 15% parotid, 5% sublingual; majority radiopaque

    85% of submandibular gland stones are in Wharton's duct

- chronic inflammatory disease

    three presentations—repeated acute episodes (normal between episodes), slow-progressive enlargement with repeated acute episodes, slow-progressive, painless enlargement (can be confused clinically with neoplasm)

    chronic recurrent sialadenitis—local or diffuse swelling, incomplete obstruction of ductal system, focal narrowing of main duct and central ductal dilatation (sialectasia), peripheral ducts and acini may not be visualized—due to destruction

- autoimmune disease

    common histology—lymphoid infiltration (BLL - benign lymphoepithelial lesion)

    classification -

        (1) recurrent parotitis (children), (2) primary Sjögren's syndrome—90% women, increased risk of lymphoma, (3) secondary Sjögren's syndrome (usually with rheumatoid arthritis)

    initially involves peripheral ducts and acini—central ducts normal at first sialogram—(characteristic) normal central system, numerous punctate collections of contrast scattered uniformly through gland; with disease progression—superimposed sialodochitis, sialadenitis

- sialosis/sialadenosis—noninflammatory, nontender parotid enlargement (usually bilateral); early—acinar hypertrophy, late—fatty atrophy

    diabetes

    chronic alcoholism (malnutrition)

    medications

- granulomatous disease

    most within juxtaglandular lymph nodes or (with parotid) in intraparotid nodes

    nontender, nonpainful, multinodular, chronic enlargement

    sarcoidosis, tuberculosis

- congenital cysts—branchial cleft or lymphoepithelial; not evident until adulthood

- acquired cysts—develop secondary to obstruction (usually intermittent or incomplete)

    termed retention cysts/mucoceles

    when in sublingual gland, termed ranulas

    no communication with ductal system on sialogram

    sialocele—saliva accumulates in cyst due to traumatic interruption of draining ducts

    multiple parotid cysts plus benign cervical adenopathy—suggests HIV infection

- ranulas—mucous retention cyst of sublingual gland

    "simple"—most common

    "deep" or "plunging"—rupture of wall of simple ranula, extends below mylohyoid muscle

---

264.3

Salivary glands—neoplasm

- the smaller the salivary gland, the greater likelihood of malignancy

Epithelial tumors

- pleomorphic adenoma = mixed tumors

    most common salivary gland tumor

    70% of all benign tumors of major salivary glands

    84% in parotid, with 90% lateral to facial nerve

    solitary, ovoid, well-demarcated

    <5% malignant

    CT—higher attenuation than parotid, do not enhance; larger lesions may be nonhomogeneous (necrosis, hemorrhage, cyst); larger tumors are lobulated

    MR—may be nonhomogeneous, intermediate SI on T_1, intermediate to high SI on T_2; moderate enhancement

- monomorphic adenoma—benign

  Warthin's tumor = adenolymphoma or papillary cystadenoma lymphomatosum

    second most common benign parotid lesion

    contains lymphoid tissue

    multiplicity, can be bilateral (30%)

    most likely of parotid tumors to undergo gross cystic change

    CT—small, homogeneous, ovoid, smoothly marginated, located in tail (superficial lobe) of parotid

    MR—more homogeneous than pleomorphic adenoma; high SI on T_2

    multiple lesions in one parotid or bilaterally—Warthin's tumor most likely diagnosis; if cystic—differential includes lymphoepithelial cysts (patients with human immunodeficiency virus [HIV])

  oncocytoma—solid tumor composed of oncocytes

    rare

    elderly patients

    parotid gland

    histologically benign

- mucoepidermoid carcinoma

    <10% of salivary tumors

    30% of malignant salivary tumors

    60% in parotid

    most common adult parotid malignancy, most common child salivary gland malignancy

    low- to high-grade, well-circumscribed to infiltrative

    Rx—surgery with wide local excision

- adenoid cystic carcinoma

    most common malignancy in submandibular gland

    4–8% of all salivary gland tumors

    slow growth rate

    prognosis worse when of minor salivary gland origin

    perineural invasion—pathologic hallmark; perineural spread—common pathway for extension

- other less common epithelial tumors—acinic cell carcinoma, squamous cell carcinoma (primary), adenocarcinoma

- metastasis—of salivary glands, parotid is most frequently involved due to intraparotid lymph nodes

Nonepithelial tumors—< 5% of salivary gland neoplasms; but > 50% in children

- hemangioma

    hemangiomas of parotid—most common salivary gland tumor in children

- lymphangioma

    benign tumor of lymphatic vessels

50% present at birth

three types—lymphangioma simplex, cavernous lymphangioma, cystic lymphangioma (= cystic hygroma)

cystic mass with thin nonvisualized wall (CT, MR)

- lymphoma

    rare—whether primary or secondary

    one or more benign-appearing masses in parotid

Miscellaneous lesions

- lipoma—1% of parotid tumors; about half within the gland, half periparotid

- neurogenic tumors—neuromas (solitary), neurofibromas (multiple) of parotid

- masseteric hypertrophy—usually bilateral

Parapharyngeal Space ....

269.11

Parapharyngeal space—basics

- difficult to examine clinically, lesions often silent clinically until quite large

- role of CT/MR—differentiation of parotid vs. extraparotid origin— determines surgical approach, and for differential diagnosis

    if parapharyngeal space fat is visible between parotid gland and posterolateral margin of mass—lesion is extraparotid

    MR > CT

        more reliable extra- vs. intraparotid distinction

        differentiation of neuromas (displace internal carotid artery [ICA] anteriorly) vs. minor salivary gland tumors (displace ICA posteriorly)

- anatomy—medial wall of parapharyngeal space = most pliable— medial bowing and downward displacement of soft palate occurs with most masses (intra- and extraparotid)

269.36–7

Parapharyngeal space—soft tissue masses (benign and malignant)

- salivary gland tumors

    most common primary lesion (50% of all primary masses) in parapharyngeal space

    80% benign mixed tumors

    prestyloid compartment of parapharyngeal space—contains retromandibular portion of parotid; tumors from this part of parotid lie anterior to ICA (thus displace ICA posteriorly)

    preserved fat plane (on axial images) between parotid and tumor of parapharyngeal space—tumor is not of parotid origin minor salivary gland tumors—arise from tissue rests in prestyloid compartment; almost all are benign pleomorphic adenomas; when large—often cystic/hemorrhagic/necrotic (heterogeneous)

- neurogenic tumors

    second most common primary lesion (25%) in parapharyngeal space

    most arise from vagus nerve (neuromas)

    when from vagus or sympathetic chain, displace ICA anteriorly (nerves lie posterior)

    most are indistinguishable from minor salivary gland tumors on CT or MR (other than by vessel displacement)

- paragangliomas

    third most common primary lesion (15%) in parapharyngeal space

    glomus vagale—most common; usually lies entirely within parapharyngeal space

    carotid body tumor—few are large enough to extend upwards into parapharyngeal space

    glomus jugulare—develop in jugular bulb (jugular fossa); spread above and below skull base usually equal in dimensions; tend to erode skull base laterally

    hypervascular; delayed scans demonstrate washout; smooth external contour

    MR—serpentine flow voids

    all three displace ICA anteriorly, with carotid body tumor also splaying internal and external carotid arteries at bifurcation

    differential diagnosis—vascular metastasis (contours irregular, invasive)

- miscellaneous

    cystic lesions—branchial cleft cyst, cystic hygroma, abscess (commonly from palatine tonsil), necrotic node

    infiltrative masses (rare)—sarcoma, lymphoma

    skull-base tumors—with extension down into parapharyngeal space; includes meningioma, chordoma, carcinoma (nasopharyngeal)

Larynx ....

271.11

Larynx

- role of radiologist—mucosal surface well-evaluated by laryngoscopy, imaging is to determine deep tumor extent and tumor margins (for the surgical decision of laryngectomy vs. voice-sparing partial resection)
- normal anatomy

    cricoid—"signet" ring of hyaline cartilage, broader "signet" portion faces posteriorly

    inferior horn of thyroid cartilage articulates laterally

    arytenoid cartilages (hyaline cartilage) articulate on upper margin posteriorly

    thyroid cartilage

double-winged, with superior and inferior horns

hyaline cartilage, thus can calcify (like cricoid and arytenoid) to variable extent

arytenoid cartilages

upper part—at level of false cord

vocal process from base—marker for level of true cord

epiglottis—fibrocartilage

hyoid bone—ceiling from which larynx is suspended; anterior body, two small superior horns (cornua), two large posterior horns

cricothyroid membrane, thyrohyoid membrane—close the gaps between cricoid and thyroid, and thyroid and hyoid; external anatomic limits of larynx

thyroarytenoid muscle—attaches to lower anterior surface of arytenoid, forms bulk of true cord; two parallel bellies—medial and lateral

pharyngeal constrictors—extend from midline raphe posteriorly, sweeping obliquely downward attaching to hyoid above and thyroid and cricoid below; lower fibers of inferior constrictor muscle given separate name = cricopharyngeus; weak point between inferior constrictor muscle and cricopharyngeus = Killian's dehiscence (Zenker's diverticula)

true cord—inferior to false cord, free margin of true cord = glottis

ventricle—recess in lateral wall of larynx between true and false cords

anterior commissure—"bare" area—laryngeal mucosa adjacent to thyroid cartilage, in midline anteriorly with each true cord attaching just slightly laterally

aryepiglottic folds—above false cords, form lateral margins of vestibule (supraglottic airspace); extend from arytenoid to lateral margin of epiglottis

pyriform sinus—lateral to aryepiglottic folds—a mucosal recess between thyroid cartilage and aryepiglottic fold

valleculae—small recesses between tongue base and free margin of epiglottis

paraglottic space—between thyroid cartilage and mucosa lining larynx

- innervation—vagus nerve (recurrent laryngeal nerve)
- lymphatic drainage

supraglottic larynx and paraglottic space lymphatics drain to upper jugular nodes

subglottic larynx lymphatics drain to paratracheal and pretracheal nodes, eventually to lower jugular nodes

---

271.11

Larynx—respiratory maneuvers, plain film, tomography

- respiratory maneuvers

quiet respiration—vocal cords off midline (slight abduction) but not completely effaced slow inspiration—true and false cords abduct, flatten, disappear

Valsalva maneuver—patient holds breath and bears down—cords adduct, angle of undersurface with lateral wall is 90°

modified Valsalva maneuver—cheeks puffed, small amount of air escaping—expands pyriform sinuses, all airway structures above true cords

phonation ("eeeee")—cords adduct

inspiratory "eeeee"—expands ventricle

- plain radiographs

low kV

variable calcification of cartilage—pitfalls (1) diagnosis of involvement by pathology from plain film, (2) "false" foreign bodies

- tomography—seldom done today (replaced by CT/MR), high-radiation dose

---

271.1211

Larynx—CT

- axial plane, 1.5–3-mm slices
- quiet breathing or breathhold
- IV contrast—tumor evaluation, but not trauma
- appearance of cartilage varies due to ossification, amount of fatty marrow
- at anterior commissure, air should abut cartilage

271.1214

Larynx—MR

- technique—sagittal T_1 localizer, coronal T_1 thin section planes perpendicular to true cord, axial T_1, axial T_2
- motion artifacts are major problem on current scanners due to long scan times (minutes)
- sagittal—assess epiglottis, valleculae, tongue base
- coronal—assess true cord (thyroarytenoid muscle within—contrasts with fat within false cord above)
- axial—assess cartilaginous erosion

271.1221

Laryngography

- rarely done today (replaced by endoscopy/imaging)
- contraindicated with significant airway obstruction
- atropine (dries up secretions), codeine (limits coughing), anesthesia (Xylocaine)
- contrast agent—oily propyliodone (Dionosil)

271.123

Larynx—barium swallow

- evaluate pharyngeal wall—motility and mucosal surface
- barium deflected around larynx (pseudomass), pyriform sinuses fill

271.14

Larynx—congenital lesions

- laryngomalacia—supraglottic, support system not firm, outgrown with age
- subglottic stenosis—narrowing (by soft tissue) from true cord level to lower cricoid, may require tracheostomy, outgrown with age
- webs

271.2

Larynx—inflammation

271.243 Croup

- inflammation of subglottic larynx
- 6 months to 3 years of age
- type 1 parainfluenza virus
- "steeple-shaped" airway (frontal film)

271.248 Epiglottitis (supraglottitis)

- swollen, cherry-red epiglottis
- older age vs. croup
- *Hemophilus influenzae*
- thickened epiglottis (lateral film)
- can progress quickly to airway compromise, patient manipulation should be minimized

271.36

Larynx—benign soft tissue neoplasm

- vocal cord nodules—due to vocal abuse, occur on free margin of vocal cord
- juvenile papillomatosis—wartlike lesions, benign, tend to recur, can involve any part of larynx
- hemangiomas

    adults—more common, usually glottic or supraglottic

    children—more likely to cause airway obstruction, usually subglottic, radiographic appearance—localized narrowing of trachea just below true cords

271.361

Larynx—cysts/laryngoceles

- cyst—can form by obstruction of mucous gland, are superficial
- laryngocele (saccular cyst)—arises from saccule or appendix of ventricle—which extends superiorly from anterior ventricle; is an enlargement of the saccule; may be air or fluid-filled; may be internal (within larynx) or external (extending through thyrohyoid membrane)

  r/o tumor at point of origin of saccule

- thyroglossal duct cyst—in infrahyoid location these are anterior outside the larynx (insinuated between strap muscles)

271.373

Larynx—squamous cell carcinoma

- general

  cancer of larynx means squamous cell (95% of malignancies of the larynx)

  cancers arise on mucosal surface

  endoscopist cannot define deep lesion extent relative to precise landmarks, this is necessary to determine if speech conserving surgery is possible

  mucosa—is realm of endoscopist

  imaging should be done before biopsy

  tumor in lymph nodes—lower rate of survival; extension outside capsule of lymph node more ominous

  voice conservation surgery: (1) supraglottic laryngectomy (supraglottic tumor)—post-surgery, patient has to relearn to swallow without aspiration, (2) vertical hemilaryngectomy (tumor confined to true cord)

  radiation therapy—speech-conserving; cartilage involvement limits use—due to radiation perichondritis, necrosis, or treatment failure

- supraglottic region—false cords, aryepiglottic folds, epiglottis

  supraglottic laryngectomy—larynx above ventricle is removed—resection line is through ventricle (landmark—midportion of arytenoid is at level of ventricle)—key to feasibility is inferior tumor extension; tumor must also be separated from anterior commissure by > 2 mm; part of one arytenoid can be removed; thyroid cartilage cannot be involved by tumor

  tumor—essentially all is squamous cell; association with ethanol and smoking

  to exclude tumor extent to true cords—on axial CT, must be a normal slice between visualization of tumor and normal cord; coronal images useful—CT/MR

  tumor isodense with muscle on CT, hyperintense with muscle on T_2 MR (thus can differentiate from thyroarytenoid muscle within true cord)

  lymph node involvement with supraglottic tumor is common; bilateral involvement also common

- glottic, infraglottic regions

  almost all lesions are squamous cell carcinoma and related to smoking

  tumors of true cord present early (hoarseness)

  applicable speech conservation surgery = vertical hemilaryngectomy: unilateral removal of true and false cords, thyroid ala

  > contraindications—extension across anterior commissure (involving posterior half of opposing true cord), subglottic extension, involvement of cricoarytenoid joint, thyroid cartilage invasion

  > key radiologically—has tumor involved cricoid (inferior extension) ?—if so, hemilaryngectomy cannot be done (cricoid forms structural foundation of larynx)

  > at anterior commissure—there is normally only mucosa between airway and thyroid cartilage; on imaging if air is opposed to cartilage, tumor is excluded

  > thyroid cartilage involvement assessed by demonstration of tumor anterior to cartilage

  > extent superiorly into false cord also prevents hemilaryngectomy

  > should assess lower neck for nodes (paratracheal, pretracheal), although nodes usually not involved in true cord lesions due to early presentation

- hypo-, laryngopharynx

  limits

  > superior—hyoid bone, valleculae

  > inferior—junction with esophagus (lower edge of cricopharyngeus, lower margin of cricoid cartilage)

  tumor in pyriform sinus can extend anteriorly to involve false cord, further extension can occur inferiorly via paraglottic space to involve true cord

  tumor in anterior wall of pharynx at level of cricoid—requires total laryngectomy

  surgical question—lower extent (pharyngoesophageal junction)—defined by barium swallow

  radiologic keys (neoplasia)—lateral involvement to surround carotid artery? posterior extension to prevertebral fascia with fixation?

  nodal spread—high jugular region

- cartilage

  tumor involvement of cricoid/thyroid: (1) disallows partial laryngectomy, (2) relative contraindication to radiation therapy

  variable ossification, tumor and unossified cartilage both have soft tissue density on CT, only reliable CT or MR sign of cartilage involvement—tumor on opposite side of cartilage from primary

271.379

Larynx—other malignant tumors

- adenocarcinoma (arising in minor salivary glands)

adenoid cystic carcinoma

mucoepidermoid

- spindle cell carcinoma—both squamous cell and spindle cell components
- sarcomas—primarily submucosal

chondrosarcoma—calcification (often ringlike)

271.4

Larynx—trauma

- most frequent—car accidents—larynx crushed against spine
- fractures of thyroid (vertical or horizontal), cricoid cartilages

cricoid fracture usually requires surgical intervention, key role of cricoid in keeping airway patent

---

271.829

Larynx—vocal cord paralysis

- superior laryngeal nerve abnormality

innervates cricothyroid muscle

arytenoid deviated toward side of lesion

look for lesion along upper vagus nerve (jugular foramen, carotid sheath)

- recurrent laryngeal nerve abnormality

innervates all larynx muscles other than cricothyroid

atrophy of thyroarytenoid muscle—cord thins, loss of subglottic angle; ventricle, pyriform sinus, vallecula enlarge ipsilaterally; cord on side of involvement does not move

look for lesion along vagus and recurrent laryngeal nerves

vagus nerve—between posterior margins of carotid artery and jugular vein

left recurrent laryngeal nerve—passes under aortic arch, then anterior and subsequently superior to lie in tracheoesophageal groove

right recurrent laryngeal nerve—passes under right subclavian artery, then anterior and subsequently superior to lie in tracheoesophageal groove

---

271.89

Larynx—miscellaneous

- Zenker's diverticulum—outpouching through inferior constrictor muscles of pharynx (most at Killian's area—between cricopharyngeus and inferior pharyngeal constictor muscles)

dehiscence is midline, but diverticulum typically protrudes to left

cricopharyngeus muscle often prominent, seen on barium swallow (posterior indentation)

- osteophytes—large anterior cervical osteophytes can cause mass effect on posterior pharyngeal wall with dysphagia
- post-therapy

    radical neck dissection—removes nodes, jugular vein, sternocleidomastoid muscle

    vertical hemilaryngectomy—soft tissue on side of resection typically absent with flat appearance; excess tissue can be present at level of cord on side of resection

    radiation changes—epiglottis thickens and arytenoids swell (this persists to some extent long-term due to fibrosis); high-radiation doses—perichondritis and chondronecrosis of cartilage

Soft Tissues of Neck ....

276.11

Soft tissues of neck

- embryology: branchial arches—four well-defined, two rudimentary; separated by branchial clefts; inner aspects of arches lined by endoderm—form four pharyngeal pouches

    branchial arches

        first (mandibular)—upper part of malleus, incus; muscles of mastication, mylohyoid, anterior belly digastric, tensor tympani and tensor veli palatini; trigeminal (V) nerve (maxillary, mandibular divisions)

        second (hyoid)—lower part of malleus, incus; styloid process; part of hyoid; stapedius, stylohyoid, posterior belly digastric, and muscles of facial expression; facial (VII) nerve

        third—part of hyoid; stylopharyngeal muscle; glossopharyngeal (IX) nerve

        fourth to sixth—thyroid, arytenoid, cricoid cartilages; pharyngeal, laryngeal muscles; vagus (X) nerve

    pharyngeal pouches

        third—thymus, inferior parathyroids

        fourth—superior parathyroids

    thyroid gland—during its descent, connected to tongue by epithelial-lined tube = thyroglossal duct; pyramidal lobe (present in 50%)—derived from lower thyroglossal duct

- division of neck into **triangles**—useful for anatomic and surgical dissection

    anterior triangle—sternocleidomastoid muscle posterolaterally and mandible superiorly; divided by hyoid bone into supra- and infrahyoid regions

        suprahyoid compartment—divided by digastric muscle

        submental triangle (paramedian)—medial to anterior belly of digastric muscle

        submandibular triangle—contains submandibular gland

    infrahyoid compartment—divided by superior belly of omohyoid muscle muscular triangle (paramedian)—bounded by superior belly of omohyoid muscle posterolaterally and sternocleidomastoid muscle laterally and posteroinferiorly; contains strap muscles, trachea, esophagus, thyroid, parathyroids, recurrent laryngeal nerves

carotid triangle—bounded by superior belly of omohyoid muscle anteroinferiorly and posterior belly of digastric superiorly; contains carotid sheath/space (carotid artery, internal jugular vein, vagus nerve)

posterior triangle—bounded by sternocleidomastoid muscle anterolaterally, trapezius posteriorly, and clavicle inferiorly; contains brachial plexus

- division of neck into **spaces**—useful for reference to axial imaging

deep cervical fascia

superficial (investing) layer—splits anteriorly to define submandibular space, splits to envelop mandible forming masticator space, splits to enclose parotid gland defining parotid space

middle layer = visceral pretracheal fascia—contains visceral space

deep layer—includes prevertebral fascia, alar fascia; prevertebral space = space between prevertebral fascia and vertebra

carotid space

posterior cervical space—posterolateral to carotid space

submandibular space—contains both sublingual (upper) and submaxillary (lower) spaces, which freely communicate

sublingual space—muscles of tongue, sublingual glands

submaxillary space—submandibular gland, nodes; an anterior extension of parapharyngeal space; infection can spread intraorally, into parapharyngeal space, or into mediastinum

parapharyngeal space—fat-filled, suprahyoid, anterior to and separated from carotid space by styloid process of temporal bone

Lymph nodes

- infrahyoid

Lateral cervical—of all cervical nodes, the most commonly involved by pathology

internal jugular—lie on outer surface of carotid sheath; includes jugulodigastric node (larger than others)—at level of hyoid bone

spinal accessory—deep to sternocleidomastoid muscle, in fat of posterior triangle

transverse cervical—at inferior aspect of posterior triangle

external jugular—superficial to sternocleidomastoid muscle

anterior cervical

prelaryngeal (delphian)

pretracheal

prethyroid

lateral tracheal (paratracheal/tracheoesophageal)

- suprahyoid

    occipital—junction of skull and neck

    mastoid—behind ear

    parotid—within and superficial to parotid gland

    submandibular—along inferior border of mandible

    facial—in subcutaneous facial tissue

    submental—between anterior bellies of digastric muscles

    sublingual

    retropharyngeal—along lateral border of longus capitis muscle

- clinical criteria

    size: >1.5 cm diameter in submandibular or jugulodigastric regions, abnormal; >1 cm diameter in other regions, abnormal; with this criteria, of abnormal nodes 80% are neoplastic, 20% hyperplastic

    imaging appearance—central lucency on CT and central high SI on T_2 or peripheral enhancement on T_1 with MR = abnormal (necrosis or tumor infiltration)

    extranodal extension—ill-defined node margins can be caused by neoplasm, inflammation, surgery, or radiation

---

276.1211

Soft tissues of neck—CT

- plane of scan should be parallel to hyoid bone and vocal cords (axial)
- IV contrast using bolus followed by rapid drip

276.1214

Soft tissues of neck— MR

- dedicated neck coil necessary

276.129

Soft tissues of neck—special exams

- phrenic nerve palsy—viral neuritis, mass (compression), trauma, surgery; nerve originates from C3–5 nerve roots, nerve lies along anterior border of anterior scalene muscle in neck, subclavian artery in thoracic inlet, and within mediastinum
- distal vagal neuropathy (= isolated recurrent laryngeal nerve palsy = hoarseness, vocal cord paralysis)—attention to carotid space (for vagus nerve) and tracheoesophageal groove (for recurrent laryngeal nerve), scan must be continued to level of aortopulmonary window for left vagal paralysis (left recurrent laryngeal nerve passes under aortic arch and then into aortopulmonary window) or to clavicle for right vagal paralysis (right recurrent laryngeal nerve loops under subclavian artery)

    differential diagnosis—inflammation, neoplasm, trauma, aortic aneurysm, left atrial enlargement

    chronic unilateral recurrent nerve palsy usually due to thyroid malignancy

- brachial plexopathy

    anatomy—formed from C5–T1 anterior nerve roots, in upper neck located adjacent to neural foramina, superior nerve roots run between anterior and middle scalene muscles, enters axilla between clavicle and first rib

    symptoms—pain, numbness, sensory and motor deficits in upper extremity

    CT—axial with intrathecal contrast

    MR—sagittal and coronal T_1s, T_2s

    differential diagnosis

    > trauma (50%)—compression, stretching, or avulsion (pseudomeningocele)

    > nontraumatic—metastases (and Pancoast tumor), radiation (radiation fibrosis has SI similar to muscle on T_1 and T_2 MR, tumors are hyperintense on T_2), nerve sheath tumors, idiopathic

---

276.14

Soft tissues of neck—congenital anomaly

276.1471 Branchial cleft anomalies

- general classification

    sinus—tract with or without a cyst, communicates with skin or gut

    fistula—communication between gut and skin

    cyst—remnant of branchial cleft or pouch

- from first branchial apparatus (5%)—can be cyst or sinus, persistent aural drainage

- from second branchial apparatus (95%)—usually cyst, mass anterior to mid- or lower portion of sternocleidomastoid muscle, most common location—lateral to internal jugular vein at level of carotid bifurcation

- present in adults, painless mass, with upper respiratory infection or trauma

- differential diagnosis—necrotic node, abscess

276.1473 Thyroglossal duct cyst

- 90% of congenital neck lesions
- more common in children than in adults
- origin—in embryo, thyroid gland develops as outgrowth from floor of pharynx = thyroglossal duct (lined with secretory epithelium), origin is at foramen cecum linguae (base of tongue); thyroid gland traverses duct to lie in front and lateral to trachea, then duct normally involutes and disappears

    caudal attachment of thyroglossal duct can persist as pyramidal lobe

    migration of thyroid can be arrested at any point (lingual thyroid = total failure of migration) fragments of thyroid tissue may lie along tract of duct even with presence of normal thyroid gland

- characteristics

  midline (75%) or off midline, most infrahyoid

  asymptomatic mass

  coexistent carcinoma <1%

  surgery—treatment of choice, since cysts can become infected; recurrence common

  differential diagnosis—laryngocele—located within cartilaginous framework of larynx

---

276.2

Soft tissues of neck—inflammation

- CT can differentiate cellulitis vs. abscess, can detect complications— venous thrombosis, airway compression, osteomyelitis
- abscess—single or multiloculated, enhancing rim; often accompanied by myositis, thickening of overlying skin, inflammation in fat
- spread of infection limited by fascial planes
- fascial spaces of neck and mediastinum are separate—with two exceptions: visceral space and prevertebral space—both communicate with mediastinum and can be route of spread for infection

---

276.23

Soft tissues of neck—AIDS

- diffuse cervical lymphadenopathy with multiple parotid cysts (lymphoepithelial cysts), nodes typically homogeneous on CT

276.23

Soft tissues of neck—tuberculosis (cervical lymphadenitis)

- tuberculous adenitis = scrofula; clinical presentation differs depending on organism, calcification in lymph nodes not specific for tuberculosis
- atypical Mycobacterium—children, involves tonsils, submandibular, parotid, preauricular, and upper cervical nodes; unilateral
- *Mycobacterium tuberculosis*—cervical lymph node involvement is manifestation of systemic disease, often bilateral posterior triangle nodes, commonly thick rim of peripheral enhancement

---

276.3

Soft tissues of neck—neoplasm

- Age distribution: children—most masses benign (inflammatory lymphadenopathy, congenital lesions), of malignant lesions—lymphoma is most common, rhabdomyosarcoma is second most common; adults—unilateral neck lesion is usually malignant (excluding thyroid disease), lymphoma is most common; > age 40—most neck masses represent metastatic disease

276.34 Lymphoma—can be unilateral or bilateral; calcification in involved nodes rare without previous chemotherapy or radiation

- Hodgkins—25%: painless neck masses (nodes), spread via lymphatic channels to contiguous node groups, extranodal involvement rare
- non-Hodgkins: frequently extranodal; three possible sites of involvement —nodal, extranodal lymphatic (Waldeyer's ring—adenoids, palatine and lingual tonsils), extranodal and extralymphatic; involvement of Waldeyer's ring with lymphoma can be difficult to differentiate from squamous cell carcinoma and infectious mononucleosis

276.362 Lymphangioma, cystic hygroma

- general classification (by size of lymphatic spaces)—all three can be found in one lesion
    lymphangioma simplex—capillary size lymphatics
    cavernous lymphangioma—dilated lymphatics
    cystic hygroma—cysts from mm to cm in diameter
- benign, nonencapsulated, arise from lymphoid tissue
- 75% in neck
- most occur in early childhood (time of greatest lymphatic development)
- painless mass, posterior triangle of neck, multiloculated
- cross-sectional imaging—without peripheral rim enhancement, can be compressed by adjacent normal soft tissue structures
- can enlarge rapidly due to hemorrhage

276.366 Dermoid cyst

- includes epidermoid (most common in neck), dermoid, teratoid cysts
- only 7% of all dermoids occur in head and neck, of these—80% in orbit, oral (sublingual, submental) or nasal regions
- midline

276.369 Paraganglioma

- types—carotid body tumor (carotid bifurcation), glomus vagale (nodose ganglion of vagus nerve), glomus jugulare (jugular ganglion of vagus nerve), glomus tympanicum (middle ear)
- carotid body tumor
    painless, slow-growing
    splays external and internal carotid arteries
    dense nonhomogeneous blush on angiography
    multiple signal voids on MR (vessels)

276.369 Lipoma

- benign, encapsulated
- more common in the obese
- can compress adjacent structures

276.37 Liposarcoma

- like lipomas, these are rare in head and neck
- combination of fat and soft tissue elements

276.375

Metastatic neoplasm

- cervical lymph node involvement in squamous cell carcinoma—carries diminished cure rate; prognosis better for solitary ipsilateral node > multiple ipsilateral > solitary contralateral > bilateral
- occult primary tumor with nodal metastases—most common sites of primary tumor include nasopharynx, pyriform sinus, tongue base, thyroid

276.431

Soft tissues of neck—vascular abnormalities (trauma)

- common pitfall—mistake internal jugular vein for mass (right usually larger than left, asymmetry in size common)
- venous thrombosis

    causes

> drug abuse
>
> central venous catheterization
>
> compression by benign/malignant disease
>
> hypercoagulable state
>
> infection

    CT—enlarged vein, enhancement of vessel wall, collateral venous channels

    ultrasound—itral echoes, lack of venous pulsations, lack of change in size with Valsalva maneuver, noncompressible

SPINE

MR Technique ....

30.121411

Spin-echo technique

- basics

    90° RF pulse followed by a 180° RF pulse

    generates signal "echo" at time TE

    pulsing repeated at intervals of TR

    T_1-weighting achieved by maximizing tissue differences due to T_1 by use of short TR, and minimizing differences due to T_2 by short TE

    T_2-weighting achieved by maximizing tissue differences due to T_2 by use of long TE, and minimizing differences due to T_1 by long TR

- T_1-weighted

    short TR, TE (< 500, < 25, respectively)—fat (including marrow) is high SI, CSF is low SI, cord, nerve roots, and disk are intermediate SI

    longer TR (1000–1500)—decreases T_1 contrast, improves SNR, increases slice coverage

    T_1 = longitudinal or spin-lattice relaxation time, time for recovery of longitudinal magnetization

    T_1—increases with magnetic field strength

    utility—anatomic detail, evaluation of contrast enhancement

- T_2-weighted

    long TR, TE (> 2000, > 45, respectively)—CSF and normal hydrated disks are high SI (long T_2), cord and nerve roots are intermediate SI, fat (including marrow) is low SI

    longer TE (> 80)—increases T_2 contrast, decreases SNR, decreases slice coverage

    longer TR (> 3000)—minimizes T_1 contrast, increases SNR

    best T_2-weighting—longer TR, TE (> 3000, > 90)

    T_2 = transverse or spin-spin relaxation time, time for magnetization in the transverse plane to dephase and lose coherence

    T_2—independent of magnetic field strength

    utility—detection and characterization of pathology, visualization of CSF

    scan times—long, due to long TR

Fast spin-echo technique

- multiple spin echoes generated following each 90° RF pulse by rapidly cycling the 180° RF pulse; = RARE (rapid acquisition with relaxation enhancement)
- when T_2-weighted—similar tissue contrast to conventional T_2 spin echo but fat is bright, also less signal loss due to susceptibility (poor depiction of hemosiderin/ferritin/deoxyhemoglobin)
- shorter acquisition time (vs. conventional spin-echo technique); scan time reduced in principle by a factor equal to number of echoes acquired

30.121412

Spoiled gradient-echo (GRE) technique (= FLASH = SP-GRASS)

- transverse magnetization is "spoiled," does not contribute to FID, longitudinal magnetization allowed to approach steady state
- no 180° pulse (definition of GRE)—echo (signal) created by gradients
- increased sensitivity to magnetic field inhomogeneities and susceptibility (T_{2*}) due to absence of 180° pulse—thus increased artifact from metal, improved detection of hemosiderin/ferritin
- TR, TE, flip (tip) angle variable—similar contrast to spin echo when 90° flip angle used, or at lower flip angles with shorter TRs

    "long" TR—500 msec

  > 10° (low) flip angle—T_2 contrast
  >
  > 90° (high) flip angle—T_1 contrast

    "short" TR—50 msec

  > less T_2 contrast at low flip angle, approaches T_1 contrast more rapidly than "long" TR as flip angle is increased
  >
  > lower SNR (vs. longer TR)
  >
  > high vessel SI due to TOF inflow enhancement

Rephased gradient-echo (GRE) technique (= FAST = GRASS)

- an SSFP (steady-state free precession) technique, uses SSFP FID
- transverse magnetization is preserved (vs. spoiled GRE)
- difference from spoiled GRE—due to degree to which SSFP echo contributes to FID—this effect increases at short TR and large flip angle— result is higher CSF SI (greatest contribution is from tissues with long T_2)
- TR, TE, flip (tip) angle variable

    "long" TR—500 msec

  > 10° (low) flip angle—T_2 contrast
  >
  > 90° (high) flip angle—T_1 contrast (except CSF, which remains intermediate SI)

    "short" TR—50 msec

  > less T_2 contrast at low flip angle (vs. long TR), approaches T_1 contrast as flip angle is increased
  >
  > typical technique employs only partial rephasing—but complete rephasing gives very high CSF SI
  >
  > lower SNR (vs. longer TR)
  >
  > high vessel SI due to TOF inflow enhancement

Image anomalies (GRE techniques)

- phase cycling

  > depending on echo time, fat signal may add (in phase) or subtract (out-of-phase) from water signal—result is large cancellation (when out-of-phase) of signal at fat-water interfaces

at 1.5 T, signals are in phase at TE = 4.3, 8.7, 13.0, . . . msec and out-of-phase at TE = 6.5, 10.9, 15.2, . . . msec

- local magnetic susceptibility effects

  reduces SI

  minimized by use of short TE and high bandwidth

  largest affect at interfaces of tissues with markedly different magnetic susceptibility, for example air-soft tissue

  produces lower SI of bone marrow on GRE techniques (vs. spin echo)

CSF visualization (high SI)

- Spin echo—requires long TR, long TE
- Fast spin echo—reduced scan time (vs. spin echo)
- GRE—low flip angle; short TR permits further scan time reduction

---

30.121413

Short tau inversion recovery (STIR)

- utility—fat suppression—dependent on TI (inversion time) choice
- contrast dependence—T_1
- pulse sequence

  180°–90°–180° RF pulsing (initial "inverting" pulse)

  short TE (< 20) to minimize T_2 contrast

  long TR (> 2000) to allow recovery of longitudinal magnetization
- tissue appearance (magnitude reconstruction)

  inverted magnetization recovers, must cross through null point (bounce point)

  suppression of signal from tissue that at time of observation has recovered to longitudinal magnetization of zero—fat has shortest T_1 and is first to pass through null point

  to null fat, proper TR and TI must be chosen, choice is field strength dependent

  high CSF SI (most negative signal, which is inverted with magnitude reconstruction)

30.121414

Chemical shift imaging

- spectral saturation (basis—different Larmor precessional frequencies of fat and water) = chemical shift selective (CHESS) = frequency selective

  can be used to produce fat only and water only images

  saturation of either fat or water signal achieved by application of a presaturation pulse (which is frequency, not spatially, selective)

  magnetic field inhomogeneities lead to varying tissue suppression across the image

30.12149

Spatial resolution, matrix size, scan time, truncation artifacts

- large pixels

    poor edge definition, poor definition of small structures

    scan time reduced and SNR improved if large pixel dimension achieved by reduction in number of phase-encoding steps

    prominent truncation artifacts (also referred to as "ringing" or "Gibbs" artifact)—with 128 matrix on sagittal T_1-weighted scans, can lead to prominent low SI stripe overlying cord (mimicking a syrinx)

- small pixels (high spatial resolution)

    achieved with larger matrix size at cost of lower SNR and longer scan time

    reduced truncation artifacts

- pixel dimensions

    determined by FOV divided by matrix size along each axis

- scan time = (number of phase-encoding steps) × (number of acquisitions) × (TR)

- truncation artifacts

    more severe at sharp boundaries between tissues of markedly different contrast

    more severe with larger pixels

Sampling bandwidth (56 Hz/pixel = extremely low, 390 Hz/pixel = extremely high)

- definition—total time allowed to acquire the signal (in digital sampling of the signal)

- low bandwidth

    increased chemical shift artifact (seen in frequency encoding = readout dimension) = misregistration between tissues containing fat vs. water

        on sagittal imaging, with frequency encoding top-to-bottom, produces asymmetry of superior vs. inferior vertebral endplates—at the interface between disk (water) and vertebral body (fat)

    accentuated magnetic field errors (field inhomogeneity, metal objects)

    improved SNR

    frequently employed on T_2-weighted studies with long TE

Field-of-view (FOV), image aliasing

- large FOV

    imaging volume lies within boundaries of encoding (no aliasing)

    larger acquisition matrix required to maintain high spatial resolution

- small FOV (with matrix size held constant)

    high spatial resolution

    reduced SNR (if FOV is halved, SNR is reduced by a factor of four—SNR is proportional to square of FOV) aliasing (wraparound) may occur

oversampling in frequency-encoding (readout) direction prevents aliasing in this axis at no cost in SNR or scan time

oversampling in phase-encoding direction increases scan time

T_1-weighted studies generally employed to achieve high spatial resolution (small FOV)—reduction in SNR can be compensated for by increasing number of scan acquisitions

Slice thickness, volume averaging, SNR

- SNR is directly proportional to slice thickness (for example, SNR is doubled if slice thickness is doubled)

- thick sections lead to loss of detail and contrast, particularly with small anatomical structures, due to volume averaging

- imaging of the spine requires thin sections (high detail), resulting in a loss in SNR, with an increase in number of scan acquisitions typically used to regain SNR

Acquisitions, imaging time, SNR

- increasing the number of scan acquisitions (signal averaging) improves SNR (SNR $\propto \sqrt{\text{number of acquisitions}}$) but lengthens scan time (scan time $\propto$ number of acquisitions)

- cost of increasing the number of scan acquisitions is thus imaging time, with this approach often taken with T_1 studies (short TR), but with T_2 studies leads to prohibitively long scans

Plane of acquisition

- with 2-D imaging, any scan plane can be acquired (sagittal, coronal, axial, oblique), this is controlled by X, Y, and Z gradient application during RF excitation—intrinsic advantage over x-ray CT

- routine use in spine of tilted axial scans, parallel to disk space—different slices may be tilted different degrees as well

Spatial presaturation (SAT pulses)

- utility

reduction of flow artifacts

SAT pulses are applied parallel to plane of acquisition (above and below)

reduction of bulk motion artifacts

SAT pulses are applied perpendicular to plane of acquisition, to void signals from moving tissue (face and neck in cervical spine, heart and lungs in thoracic spine, anterior abdomen in lumbar spine)

- principles

used to reduce magnitude of unwanted signal

implemented by preceding the RF pulses used for imaging by a spatially selective RF pulse applied to the region producing the artifact

repeated each TR

prevents growth of longitudinal magnetization in applied area reduces total number of slices which can be acquired (requires time within scan sequence)

increases specific absorption rate (SAR)

CSF-related artifacts

- problem

    CSF flow/pulsation produces artifacts on T_2-weighted scans (when CSF is of high SI) which can obscure visualization of structures within the spinal canal (motion in any direction manifests itself as artifact in the phase-encoding direction if uncorrected)

- solution (artifact reduction)

    gradient moment nulling (= flow compensation = motion artifact suppression technique (MAST) = gradient motion refocusing)

    additional gradient pulses are incorporated into the scan technique to eliminate phase errors

    minimizes contribution of motion which occurs during time TE

    applicable to most MR scan techniques

    correction can be for velocity (first order), acceleration (second order), or higher orders of motion—most techniques compensate only for velocity

    correction can be in one, two, or three axes—most techniques correct in readout, or readout and slice select directions

    implementation increases minimum TE which can be achieved with a scan technique

    electrocardiogram (ECG) triggering

    data collection synchronized with cardiac cycle

    minimizes contribution of motion which occurs between successive TR intervals

    implementation restricts choice of TR

Phase, frequency-encoding directions

- pulsation/motion artifacts are observed in phase-encoding direction

    origin

    data acquisition is repeated for each phase-encoding step (typically 256 times, over a scan duration of 5 to 10 min)—each data acquisition thus possesses error due to motion which occurs between steps

    these signal errors, regardless of direction of motion, then mismapped in phase-encoding direction

- orientation of encoding can be selected to reduce artifact across region of interest (swapping phase and frequency axes changes direction of artifact)

- choice of axis may be restricted by wraparound (necessity of choosing frequency axis to prevent image aliasing)

3-D imaging

- no gap between slices (vs. 2-D imaging)
- third dimension is phase-encoded

- for reasonable scan times, very short TRs must be used (thus GRE techniques with low RF flip angles)
- permits multiplanar reformatting (MPR)—reconstruction of high resolution images in any arbitrary plane
- volume and surface rendering of structures possible

Coils

- whole-body (RF transmission and reception)
    good signal uniformity across FOV
    poor SNR vs. surface coils
    large imaging volume (tissue coverage)
- surface (RF reception)
    rapid signal drop-off (nonuniform signal across FOV)
    high SNR (in close proximity to coil)
    limited imaging volume—typically only cervical, thoracic, or lumbar spine can be covered in any one scan acquisition
    routinely used for all spine imaging, due to high SNR

Linear vs. circular polarization

- circularly polarized (CP) surface coils have superior SNR (superior image quality) to linearly polarized (LP) surface coils of similar configuration
- theory of operation
    transverse component of magnetization is what is detected as signal in MR
    transverse component is comprised of two fields, oriented at 90°
    LP antenna detects only one of these two components
    CP antenna detects both components simultaneously—40% theoretical improvement in SNR

Myelography Technique ....

30.122

Terminology/imaging appearance

- block—displaced sac with obliterated subarachnoid space and cord compression
- lesion localization
    extradural mass—compression of thecal sac
    intradural extramedullary mass—filling defect, outlined by sharp meniscus of contrast, ipsilateral subarachnoid space enlarged up to mass, spinal cord deviated away from mass
    intramedullary mass—smooth cord enlargement, gradual subarachnoid space effacement

Cervical Spine...

31.1214

Normal cervical spine

- Anatomy
  - seven cervical vertebral bodies, eight cervical nerves
    - C1—atlas, a bony ring
    - C2—axis, with dens extending superiorly
    - C3–C7—gradual increase in size of vertebral body as progress caudally
  - uncinate process—bilateral superior projections from C3–C7 which indent disk and vertebral body above (posterolaterally), forming uncovertebral joints
  - transverse foramen—within transverse process, contains vertebral artery
  - normal slight increase in spinal cord size at C4–6
  - neural foramina course anterolaterally at 45° angle with slight inferior course—oblique to sagittal and axial imaging planes
  - prominent epidural venous plexus, sparse epidural fat (vs. lumbar region)
  - dermatomes—hand innervated by C6 (thumb), C7 (middle finger), and C8 (little finger)
- T_1-weighted spin-echo imaging
  - fat (vertebral body marrow)—high SI, cord and disks—intermediate SI (on high-quality images, gray and white matter within the cord can be distinguished on the basis of SI), CSF—low SI
  - sagittal images—neural foramina poorly visualized due to oblique orientation
  - short scan time, high SNR, high spatial resolution
  - utility—detection of structural abnormalities, marrow infiltration, degenerative disease, contrast enhancement (gadolinium chelates)
- T_2-weighted spin-echo imaging
  - CSF and hydrated disks—high SI, cord and soft tissues—intermediate SI, fat (vertebral body marrow)—intermediate to low SI
  - current standard technique—dual echo ECG or pulse triggered spin echo
  - above technique is being replaced by fast spin echo, due to shorter scan time and less sensitivity to motion artifacts (especially CSF pulsation)
  - utility—detection of spinal cord abnormalities (edema, gliosis, demyelination, neoplasia), evaluation of thecal sac dimensions (canal compromise)
- gradient-echo imaging (low flip angle, T_2-weighted)
  - CSF and disks—high SI, cord—intermediate SI, marrow—low SI (due to magnetic susceptibility effects); good gray-white matter differentiation within cord
  - standard technique for axial cervical spine imaging

utility—myelographic-like sagittal and axial images, detection of degenerative disease (disk herniation, canal compression, foraminal stenosis), evaluation of intrinsic cord abnormalities—in axial plane (multiple sclerosis [MS], tumors, edema, hemorrhage)

may slightly exaggerate canal and foraminal stenosis due to susceptibility effects

Normal vascular anatomy

- spinal arteries—one anterior (supplies 70% of cord), two posterior (supply 30% of cord)

    cervical—anterior spinal artery supplied by several radicular arteries

    thoracolumbar—anterior spinal artery = artery of Adamkiewicz

31.125

Flexion and extension views

- MR—can be acquired with rapid imaging

    T_1—reduced number of phase-encoding steps

    T_2—fast-spin echo technique

    range of motion limitation likely, based on surface coil choice

- utility

    demonstration of spinal cord compression (MR) not seen in neutral position (rheumatoid arthritis)

    evaluation of potential instability

        trauma

        chronic inflammatory diseases (atlanto-occipital atlantoaxial levels)

31.12988

IV-contrast media—normal-enhancing structures

- venous plexus

    external vertebral plexus—network of veins along anterior vertebral body, laminae, and spinous, transverse, and articular processes

    internal vertebral plexus—network of veins in epidural space, both anteriorly and posteriorly

        anterior plexus—larger, with longitudinal veins on each side of posterior longitudinal ligament, tapers at disk space level, displacement and engorgement often accompany disk herniation

    all drain via intervertebral veins which accompany spinal nerves within foramina

31.142 (see also 33.142)

Spinal stenosis

- congenital

    cause—(cervical spine) short pedicles

> may be underlying syndrome—Down's, achondroplasia
>
> symptoms—myelopathic—extremity weakness, gait abnormalities, reflex changes, muscle atrophy
>
> dimensions
>
> > relative spinal stenosis—≤ 13 mm canal diameter—may be symptomatic
> >
> > absolute spinal stenosis—< 10 mm
>
> predisposed to
>
> > earlier, more severe degenerative changes
> >
> > traumatic spinal cord injury

- degenerative (acquired)
  - cause—advanced degenerative disk disease = spondylosis
    - contributing factors
      - decreased disk height with thickening, buckling of intraspinal ligaments
      - calcification of posterior longitudinal ligament, ligamentum flavum
      - disk bulges, herniations, osteophytic spurs (anteriorly)
      - hypertrophy of facet joints (posteriorly)
  - symptom onset—middle age, elderly (older population than that affected by disk herniation, with some overlap)
  - symptoms—myelopathic—progressive/intermittent numbness, weakness upper extremities, pain, abnormal reflexes, muscle wasting (interosseous muscles of hand), staggering gait
  - dimensions (anteroposterior—most accurately measured on axial images)
    - normal > 13 mm
    - borderline 10—13 mm (may experience symptoms)
    - < 10 mm—diagnostic of stenosis
  - most commonly affected levels—C4–5, C5–6, C6–7 (multilevel involvement common)
  - imaging appearance
    - mild disease—ventral subarachnoid space is effaced
    - severe disease—cord flattening, impingement, and/or myelomalacia (edema, gliosis, cystic change)
- neuroforaminal (uncovertebral joint spurring)
  - uncovertebral joints = joints of Luschka
    - along posterolateral margins of cervical vertebral bodies
    - uncinate process extends superiorly to articulate with a depression in inferior endplate of adjacent vertebral body
    - present from C3 to C7, thus can cause foraminal narrowing from C2–3 to C6–7
    - hypertrophic spurs—narrow the anteromedial part of neural foramen
      - combined with disk space narrowing (decreased height of neural foramen)—cause nerve root compression (more common cause of radiculopathy than disk herniation)

due to anterolateral (and slight inferior) course of neural foramen, oblique imaging gives best demonstration of foramina

---

31.1432

Klippel-Feil syndrome

- fusion of two or more cervical vertebrae, most commonly C2–3 and C5–6—at affected levels, intervertebral disk absent
- 50% demonstrate classic triad—short neck, low posterior hairline, limited neck motion
- common associated anomalies—deafness, congenital heart disease, Sprengel's deformity (elevation and rotation of the scapula), urologic abnormalities; may have (uncommonly associated) syringomyelia, diastematomyelia
- types

    I—extensive cervical, thoracic fusion

    II—one or two cervical fusions—most common, may have associated hemivertebrae, atlanto-occipital fusion

    III—type I or II with additional lower thoracic, lumbar fusions
- clinical

    often asymptomatic

    can have cord and nerve root compression

    predisposed to spinal cord injury with minor trauma

    potential instability of unfused segments (predisposed to hypermobility at these levels)

31.1473

Abnormalities involving cerebellar tonsils

- ectopia

    position best evaluated on sagittal images (MR)

    mild inferior displacement seen in asymptomatic normal individuals —majority of normal cases, tonsils lie above foramen magnum—but may lie as far as 5 mm below and still be normal

    retain normal globular configuration
- Chiari I malformation

    tonsils pointed or wedge-shaped, low-lying

    associated findings—syrinx, craniovertebral junction abnormalities (basilar impression, occipitalization of atlas, Klippel-Feil syndrome)

    normal position of fourth ventricle

    best evaluated by MR

    clinical—variable

        asymptomatic (usual)

        symptoms related to brainstem compression (headache, cranial nerve deficits, nystagmus, ataxia) or cervical syrinx (extremity weakness, hyperreflexia, central cord syndrome) symptoms related to extension of syrinx into medulla (rare, = syringobulbia)—hemifacial numbness, facial pain, vertigo, dysphagia, loss of taste

symptomatic patients may benefit from decompression of foramen magnum or shunting of syrinx

- Chiari II malformation

most common major malformation of posterior fossa

nearly always associated with hydrocephalus and myelomeningocele

findings

brain—low insertion of tentorium cerebelli (small posterior fossa), hypoplastic tentorium cerebelli (large incisura)—towering cerebellum, extension of cerebellum around the brainstem (laterally/anteriorly), flattened pons with scalloping of clivus and petrous bones, prominent prepontine CSF space, elongated midbrain, small elongated slitlike fourth ventricle (10% "ballooned" or trapped), fusion of colliculi (beaking of quadrigeminal plate/ tectum), fenestration of falx (interdigitation of cerebral gyri), agenesis of corpus callosum, large massa intermedia

spine—displacement of brainstem and hypoplastic cerebellum into upper cervical canal, cervicomedullary kinking (medulla and cervical cord overlap), enlarged foramen magnum and upper cervical canal, smaller C1 ring with compression of displaced brainstem and cerebellar tonsils and cerebellar vermis, bifid C1 arch, posterior arch defects—C3 to C7, syringomyelia (can occur in any location, more commonly low cervical, thoracic)

- Chiari III malformation—rare—osseous defect of occiput and upper cervical spine, cerebellar herniation into cervico-occipital encephalocele

---

31.1475

Basilar invagination

- definition—location of tip of odontoid 5 or more mm above Chamberlain's line (drawn from posterior margin of hard palate to posterior lip of foramen magnum)
- secondary (acquired) types = basilar impression—seen with osteomalacia, osteoporosis, fibrous dysplasia, Paget's disease, achondroplasia, osteogenesis imperfecta
- often associated with fusion of atlas and occiput (occipitalization/ assimilation)

Platybasia

- angle formed by the clivus and floor of anterior cranial fossa > 140° (normal 125° to 140°)
- can accompany basilar invagination

31.1476

Os odontoideum

corticate ovoid ossicle, distinct from body of C2

etiology—controversial—ascribed to both congenital and acquired causes

must be distinguished from fracture of dens (not uncommon following major trauma)

31.1831

Neurofibromatosis

- type 1

    chromosome 17, autosomal dominant

    clinical presentation

        café-au-lait spots

        iris hamartomas (Lisch nodules)

    findings (spine)—scoliosis, patulous dural sac, meningoceles, neurofibromas of exiting roots

- type 2

    chromosome 22, autosomal dominant (much less common than type 1)

    findings

        brain

            bilateral acoustic neuromas (characteristic)

            schwannomas, gliomas, hamartomas

        spine

            intradural lesions

                extramedullary—neurofibromas, meningiomas

                intramedullary—ependymomas, low-grade astrocytomas

- spine manifestations (types 1 and 2)

    bony dysplasia, dural ectasia, lateral meningoceles

    cord (infrequent with neurofibromatosis, type 1) and extradural lesions

    peripheral nerve lesions—may be solitary, or involve multiple nerves in plexiform manner (with enlargement over a considerable length)

- MR—neurofibromas characteristically are markedly hyperintense on T_2

von Hippel-Lindau syndrome

- autosomal dominant syndrome, with renal carcinoma, pheochromocytoma, cysts of kidney and pancreas
- hemangioblastomas of cerebellum and spinal cord
- multiple hemangioblastomas considered diagnostic

31.22

Sarcoidosis

- noncaseating granulomatous disease of unknown etiology
- CNS involved clinically in 5%

most common sites of involvement—basal leptomeninges, floor of third ventricle

spinal cord involvement—much less common—fusiform cord enlargement, nodular parenchymal enhancement (broad-based along cord surface), thin pial enhancement

treatment—steroids—follow-up scans may demonstrate return to normal appearance

---

31.242

Epidural abscess

- etiology—hematogenous spread, direct extension, penetrating trauma
- *Staphylococcus aureus*—most common organism
- thickened inflamed tissue initially, progressing to frank abscess (liquid center)

    enhancement (MR) can be homogeneous, or rimlike with central low SI (pus)

- may cause cord compression (due to inflammation, granulation tissue, fluid)

31.3113

Osteochondroma = osteocartilaginous exostosis

- bony excrescence, with cartilaginous-covered cortex, medullary cavity contiguous with parent bone
- 8% of primary bone tumors, one-third of benign tumors
- rare in spine

    cervical spine location most common (one-half)

    spinous or transverse process involved

31.3183

Aneurysmal bone cyst

- benign, non-neoplastic
- multiloculated, expansile, highly vascular, osteolytic
- often contains blood degradation products
- 80% less than age 20
- 20% in spine (cervical and thoracic spine most common)

    majority in posterior elements

31.33 (see also 32.33, 33.33)

Cervical metastases

- background (vertebral body metastases)

    major source of morbidity in cancer patients

    vertebrae involved in up to 40% of patients dying of metastatic disease may cause bone expansion, pathologic fractures

plain films—insensitive for detection (at least 50% of the bone must be destroyed)

bone scans—high sensitivity, low specificity (false positives—infection, trauma, degenerative disease)

CT—limited extent of coverage, poor soft tissue evaluation

myelography—cord compression can be evaluated, but lesions are inferred (not directly visualized)

MR—high sensitivity and specificity, excellent coverage, excellent soft tissue evaluation

- MR appearance

low SI on T_1 (replacing high SI normal marrow)

often high SI on T_2; blastic metastases low SI on T_2

enhance (often to isointensity with normal marrow) following IV-contrast administration; enhancement useful for improved definition of epidural extent

- high cervical lesions—high morbidity—extensive sensory and motor deficits, spread to skull base may cause cranial neuropathies
- squamous cell carcinoma of neck—spreads by local invasion, involvement of cervical spine and skull base not uncommon

31.3631 (see also 32.3631)

Astrocytoma

- most common intramedullary tumor in cervical region
- lower incidence in distal spinal cord (opposite of ependymomas)
- peak incidence—third and fourth decades
- grade—tends to be lower than for brain astrocytomas
- imaging appearance

fusiform dilatation of spinal cord

long segment of involvement, near complete involvement of width of cord

decreased SI on T_1, increased SI on T_2

enhancement typical, but not invariable

31.365

Arteriovenous malformation

- see 32.365

31.3651

Hemangioblastoma

- imaging features

enhancing, highly vascular, intramedullary nodule

intramedullary cyst (nonCSF SI)—cyst wall does not enhance

cord enlargement (edema)

enlarged draining veins

- most frequently found in posterior fossa, much less common in cord (of these, 40% cervical spine and 50% thoracic spine)
- can be solitary or multiple, latter associated with von Hippel-Lindau disease

---

31.3661 (see also 32.3661)

Meningioma

- 25% of intraspinal tumors, second in incidence to neurinomas
- usually solitary
- peak age incidence—45 years
- histologically benign, slow-growing, cause symptoms due to cord and nerve root compression
- intense enhancement
- 1–3% at foramen magnum—of lesions here, three-fourth are meningiomas, one-fourth neurofibromas

---

31.368

Syringohydromyelia

- longitudinally oriented fluid cavities within spinal cord

  syringobulbia (subset)—extension into brainstem

  etiology

  obstruction of CSF flow at foramen magnum (usually due to Chiari II malformations)—slitlike in appearance

  extension of syrinx superiorly to involve brainstem—tubular/saccular in appearance—result of episodes of increased intra-abdominal pressure (coughing, sneezing)

  symptoms—facial pain and numbness, dysphagia, vertigo, loss of taste, respiratory problems (in severe cases)

- pathologic definitions (these two entities are indistinguishable on imaging)

  syringomyelia—cavity which is separate from but may communicate with central canal

  hydromyelia—dilatation of central canal, lined by ependymal cells

- imaging

  sagittal plane—to define extent

  axial plane—necessary to evaluate/detect small cavities

- etiology

  trauma (may develop over years after event)

  neoplasm

  arachnoiditis

  surgery

  Chiari I, II malformations

- symptoms (cervical syrinx)

    progressive upper extremity weakness, muscle wasting

    decreased upper extremity reflexes

    loss of pain, temperature sensation; preservation of light touch, proprioception

    enlarging syrinx in post-traumatic patient can cause neurologic deterioration

    treatment—shunting into subarachnoid, pleural, or peritoneal space

---

31.369

Cavernous angioma

- one of four vascular malformations (capillary telangiectasia, cavernous angioma, venous angioma, arteriovenous malformation [AVM])
- angiographically occult, thus together with capillary telangiectasia (which most commonly are solitary, occur in pons, and are clinically silent) form the group of occult cerebrovascular malformations
- can occur anywhere in CNS, multiple in one third, 80% familial, most asymptomatic although seizure a common clinical presentation
- imaging features

    small, smoothly marginated

    border (rim)—mildly hypointense on T_1, markedly hypointense on T_2 (hemosiderin/ferritin within macrophages that have phagocytosed blood)

    centrally—honeycomb of vascular spaces separated by fibrous stands (mixture of high and low SI on T_2)

31.37 (see also 32.37, 33.37)

Metastases (within thecal sac)

- spinal cord metastasis

    5% of metastatic disease to CNS will have intramedullary spinal metastases

    thoracic cord most often involved

    bronchogenic carcinoma—most often primary

    imaging features—enhancing focus with surrounding cord edema
- leptomeningeal metastases

    most sensitive imaging modality—contrast-enhanced MR (superior to CT myelography, which cannot detect intramedullary tumor involvement)

    imaging appearance (cervical)

        soft tissue nodules (within thecal sac)

        irregular cord surface contour (tumor adherent to or encasing cord)

        thin coating of spinal cord (especially dorsal aspect)

    may demonstrate contrast enhancement (MR)

entire spinal axis (cervical, thoracic, lumbar) should be studied to rule out disease—with attention to lumbar region (effect of gravity)

31.4

Mechanisms of spine injury

- flexion—anterior wedging, vertebral body fractures

    severe injury—disruption of posterior longitudinal ligament and interspinous ligaments, facet distraction, anteroposterior subluxation

- extension—posterior element fracture

    severe injury—anterior longitudinal ligament rupture, subluxation

- axial loading (vertical compression, from diving or jumping accidents)—vertebral body compression (burst) fractures, lateral element fractures

- rotation (rarely isolated, usually occurs with flexion-extension injury)—lateral mass fractures, facet subluxations

Imaging in spine trauma

- high resolution CT with multiplanar reconstruction—for evaluation of bone
- MR—for evaluation of cord and soft tissues

Findings in spine injury

- patterns of acute injury to spinal cord (MR, T_2)

    Type I—central hypointensity with thin rim of hyperintensity (deoxyhemoglobin with methemoglobin periphery)—very poor prognosis (little neurologic recovery)

    Type II—uniform hyperintensity (spinal cord edema)—excellent prognosis (substantial neurologic recovery, often complete)

    Type III—isointense centrally with thick rim of hyperintensity (combination of hemorrhage and edema)—variable course, some recovery of function

- myelomalacia—describes findings with cord compression

    early stage

    > cord edema—compression and stasis within venules, blood-cord barrier disruption
    >
    > T_2—high SI

    intermediate stage

    > cystic necrosis within central gray matter
    >
    > T_2—high SI, T_1—low SI

    chronic stage

    > progressive cystic degeneration centrally—may result in a syrinx
    >
    > > presence and extent of syrinx best defined on axial T_1 images (sagittal images—have potential partial volume problems)
    >
    > cord atrophy may be present—defined as cord diameter of < 6 mm in cervical region, < 5 mm in thoracic region

- post-traumatic disk herniation

    most common in cervical spine (vs. thoracic or lumbar)

may occur following minor trauma (cervical)

incidence increases with severity of trauma

most common with hyperextension injury, and at C5–6

acceleration hyperextension = whiplash

acute posterolateral disk herniations prevalent

symptoms—immediate neck and arm pain

in patients with cervical fractures, disk herniation is most common immediately below fracture

- extradural hematoma
- CT vs. MR

    CT superior for demonstration of osseous injury

    MR superior for demonstration of cord injury and traumatic disk herniation

- MR-scan technique

    T_2-weighted images important for demonstration of marrow edema (vertebral body microfractures) and soft tissue injury

Specific osseous injuries

- atlanto-occipital dislocation

    distance between dens to basion (anterior margin of foramen magnum) should not be > 12.5 mm on lateral film

    often fatal

- Jefferson fracture

    burst fracture involving both anterior and posterior arches of C1 (atlas)

    unless transverse ligament is disrupted, patient is neurologically intact

    may be unstable

- Dens fracture

    occurs with both hyperflexion and hyperextension

    classification—by anatomic location of fracture line

    type I—involves upper dens

    type II—involves junction of dens and body, most common type of injury, highest rate of nonunion

    type III—extends into C2 body

    transverse fracture may be inapparent on axial images

- Hangman's fracture

    due to hyperextension

    bilateral neural arch fractures of C2

- Clay-Shoveler's fracture (flexion injury)—avulsed spinous process, usually C6 or C7

31.413

Flexion-rotation injury

- abnormalities are attributable to combination of flexion and rotation bilateral facet fractures/dislocation—flexion

unilateral facet fracture—flexion plus rotation

vertebral body compression fractures—flexion

injury to posterior musculature, ligaments—flexion; unilaterality—rotation

- MR is preferred for evaluation of the cord (applicable to all trauma)
- CT is preferred for evaluation of posterior element fractures and canal narrowing due to retropulsed fragments (applicable to all trauma)

31.429

Perched facet

- plain film—may be suboptimal for lower cervical spine
- CT—misalignments of facets may be inapparent unless sagittal reconstructions performed
- MR—direct sagittal views well-delineate vertebral and facet alignment

---

31.452

Surgery for cervical spondylosis

- preoperatively—damage to cord results from chronic compression with ischemia
- aim of surgery—to prevent further deterioration
- surgical approach

    anterior—for one or two level stenosis

        most common neurosurgical procedure in cervical disk disease

        procedure

            diskectomy with bone graft placed to achieve stable fusion, portions of adjacent vertebral bodies may or may not be removed

            SI characteristics of graft—variable

            > 2 years following surgery, continuous marrow SI is seen at site of fusion (no evidence of bone graft or native disk)

        propensity to develop (long-term) new herniation above or below site of fusion

    posterior (laminectomy)—for congenital narrowing or extensive contiguous disease (multiple levels)

- MR findings

    T_2 high SI in cord postoperatively—can be due to gliosis (present preoperatively) or postoperative complications (cord contusion, infarction)

31.47

Radiation therapy changes

- confined to treatment area ("port")

- uniform fatty replacement of bone marrow—occurs as early as 2 weeks following initiation of therapy, with temporal progression
- imaging—sagittal T_1 spin echo recommended

31.492

Brachial plexus injury

- possible end results

    post-traumatic neuroma

    fibrosis

    meningocele—with or without nerve root avulsion

    MR—lesion follows course of nerve root in foramen, with CSF SI on all sequences

- nerve root avulsion—best evaluated by myelography

31.663 (and 32.33)

Eosinophilic granuloma

- benign, non-neoplastic
- lytic lesion without surrounding sclerosis
- classic cause of vertebra plana (single collapsed vertebral body)

31.71

Rheumatoid arthritis

- synovitis, can occur in any synovial-lined joint
- in axial skeleton, upper cervical spine most commonly involved—usually at articulation of atlas and dens

    increased distance between atlas and dens—due to subluxation (instability)

    erosion of dens (by surrounding inflammatory pannus)

    retrodental soft tissue mass (involvement of transverse ligament)

    settling of skull on atlas

- cord compression (possible complication)

31.77

Hypertrophic endplate spurs

- symptoms

    may be asymptomatic

    may mimic disk herniation

    radiographic findings may not correlate well with symptoms

- etiology

    end result of disk bulge or herniation

    during healing, bone laid down on elevated ligamentous attachments (result—spurs)

- imaging—can distinguish osteophyte from acute disk

  MR—gradient echo (T_2) images useful—disk material is high SI, spurs are very low SI (CSF outlines spurs well); postcontrast T_1 SE—enhancement of epidural venous plexus may outline low SI of spur

---

31.783 (see also 32.783, 33.783)

Disk herniation—cervical

- Cervical spine is most mobile at C4–5, C5–6, C6–7—thus level of most disk herniations
- age of presentation—third and fourth decades
- choice of exam—MR and postmyelography CT equivalent (sensitivity)

  on GRE MR, thin rim of low SI along posterior aspect of disk herniation = dura and posterior longitudinal ligament
- acute disk herniation

  symptoms

      radicular—posterolateral or foraminal herniations (compressing exiting nerve root)

      myelopathic—large central herniation

  imaging technique

      sagittal and axial planes required (MR)

      GRE (T_2) of high value in axial plane

      postcontrast T_1—enhancement of surrounding dilated epidural venous plexus (which is otherwise isointense with disk material); improves visualization of neural foramina

  imaging appearance

      anterior epidural soft tissue mass

      contiguous with disk space (unless disk fragment)

      similar SI on T_1 and T_2 to native disk
- "hard disk"—result of longstanding herniation

  covered above and below by bone spurs from endplates (due to bone remodeling—elevation of periosteum by disk herniation results in bone deposition)

  myelopathic symptoms more common (vs. radicular symptoms with acute disk herniation)

31.811

Ossification of the posterior longitudinal ligament

- uncommon cause of acquired spinal stenosis (more common etiologies are ligamentous and facet joint hypertrophy)
- more common in Orientals
- patient at risk for traumatic spinal cord injury
- multilevel involvement
- very low SI on both T_1 and T_2 (may contain centrally intermediate to high SI—marrow)

31.871

Multiple sclerosis (MS)

- imaging appearance (spinal cord plaques, MR)

    abnormal high T_2 SI with or without cord enlargement

        cord enlargement = swelling—acute disease

        edema (if present)—flame-like above and below lesion

            symptomatic (active) lesions may or may not demonstrate substantial surrounding edema

    cord lesions best detected on scans with intermediate T_2-weighting (TE = 40–50 msec)

    contrast enhancement (T_1)—active lesions

    lesions are haphazard in distribution, both in cross-section and longitudinally, disregarding anatomical boundaries; tend to be elliptical in shape, with greatest dimension along craniocaudal axis

    cord atrophy (focal or generalized)—longstanding disease

    not all patients with spinal cord lesions will demonstrate characteristic brain lesions

- histologic appearance—multifocal sharply marginated areas of demyelination

- symptoms

    recurrent focal neurologic attacks, progressive deterioration, ultimately permanent neurologic dysfunction

    decreased vibration and position sense

    weakness of one or more extremities

    disorders of micturition

    optic neuritis

- differential diagnosis

    acute transverse myelitis (multiple cord lesions, combined with characteristic brain lesions, favors MS)

31.872

Acute transverse myelitis

- imaging appearance—abnormal cord with high T_2 SI and fusiform enlargement, commonly extends over multiple segments

- symptoms—sudden loss of sensory and motor function, segmental distribution

- pathogenesis unknown

    possible etiologies—viral, vascular, autoimmune

31.9

Scan interpretation

- need for consistent, thorough approach to scan interpretation

- cerebellar tonsils, thyroid, facet joints (perched facets), and soft tissues (lymphadenopathy) deserve particular attention, as disease is common and often overlooked in these areas

Thoracic Spine ....

32.1214

Normal thoracic spine

- Anatomy
    - twelve thoracic vertebral bodies
    - ribs articulate with vertebrae both at disk and at transverse process (latter for only T1–T10)
    - exit foramina for basivertebral veins seen posteriorly within midvertebral body
    - epidural fat prominent posterior to thecal sac
- MR technique
    - coronal saturation pulse (presaturation slab) necessary to eliminate motion artifacts from chest wall and heart
    - 3-mm maximum slice thickness recommended in all planes
    - focal signal loss within CSF on T_2-weighted scans not uncommon (pulsatile CSF)

32.1221

Pantopaque (iophendylate)

- early contrast agent for myelography (no longer in use)
- oily, not water-soluble
- not unusual to leave a small amount within thecal sac following completion of myelogram—which persists for years
- occasionally now seen in older patients, free within thecal sac or trapped within root sleeve
- imaging characteristics
    - extremely x-ray dense
    - short T_1 and T_2 (high SI on T_1, low SI on T_2)

32.1453

Lateral meningocele

- protrusion (laterally) of dura and arachnoid through an enlarged neural foramen (pedicles, lamina may be thinned, dorsal surface of vertebral body scalloped)
- 85% in neurofibromatosis (thoracic paraspinal masses in neurofibromatosis more likely to be meningoceles than neurofibromas)
- most right-sided, single foramen, upper thoracic (T3–T7)
- most asymptomatic
- MR—CSF SI

32.21

Osteomyelitis

- symptoms

    often insidious

    delay in treatment dramatically increases morbidity

- pathogenesis

    children—hematogenous spread of bacteria to vascularized disk

    adult—hematogenous spread to more vascular endplate, disk involved secondarily

- imaging appearance

    plain film—frequently unremarkable until late in disease

    MR

        sensitivity > radionuclide scintigraphy

        abnormal low SI on T_1, high SI on T_2 within vertebral body (= edema, inflammatory changes)

        enhancing paraspinous and epidural soft tissue mass

        involvement of disk—distinguishes process from metastatic disease

32.23

Tuberculous spondylitis

- symptoms

    more indolent clinical course than pyogenic infection

- pathogenesis

    uncommon in US except in immigrants (Southeast Asia, South America) and immunocompromised patients

- imaging appearance

    abnormal marrow SI (within two or more adjacent vertebral bodies), cortical bone destruction, epidural soft tissue

        50% with three or more levels involved

        "skip" lesions common

    distinguishing features from pyogenic infection—relative sparing of disk, large epidural mass

    often spreads along anterior longitudinal ligament, involving multiple contiguous vertebral bodies

    epidural component—typically prevertebral, but can extend into spinal canal

    longstanding disease

        extensive bone destruction

        gibbus deformity (vertebral collapse with anterior wedging)

        cord compression (due to angulation or soft tissue mass)

- plain film, CT

    both depict extensive bone destruction and soft tissue (paraspinous) mass

- MR

    superior depiction of vertebral and paravertebral involvement compared to other modalities

    with effective therapy, return to normal in T_1 and T_2 SI of vertebral bodies, and decrease in abnormal enhancement of paravertebral soft tissue

---

32.29

Acquired immunodeficiency syndrome (AIDS)-related infection

- may present as polyradiculopathy or myelopathy
- viral etiology

    direct—cytomegalovirus, herpes simplex virus (type 2), varicella-zoster virus, toxoplasmosis

    indirect—postinfectious demyelination, parainfectious vasculitis

- differential diagnosis—neoplasm—lymphoma

32.33 (see also 31.33, 33.33)

Thoracic metastases

- MR appearance

    T_1-weighted scans—highest sensitivity for vertebral body metastases (malignant lesions, with increased cellularity, are low SI vs. normal high SI marrow fat)

    with tumors that spread via lymphatics (for example, carcinoid), important to scrutinize lateral sagittal images (and axial scans) for retroperitoneal lymphadenopathy

- sensitivity—MR well-established as more sensitive than radionuclide bone scanning (MR may detect lesions despite normal bone scan)
- specificity—degenerative changes, infection, fractures can result in false positive bone scan; MR provides higher level of discrimination (benign vs. malignant)
- epidural metastatic disease

    propensity for development with myeloma, prostate, and renal cell carcinoma

    higher incidence (however) with lung carcinoma, the most common cause of metastatic disease to vertebral column

    symptoms—epidural cord compression

        prodromal phase—central back pain (at level of disease)

        compressive phase—neurologic deficits, which begin with motor impairment (anterior cord compression)

            conus lesions—autonomic dysfunction may occur without sensory or motor deficits

    sensitivity

        without cord compression, MR superior to myelography

        with cord compression, MR = myelography

32.34

Lymphoma

- spinal involvement in 15%
- paravertebral, vertebral, and epidural lesions occur
    spinal lymphoma is most commonly caused by local spread from retroperitoneal nodes (thus paravertebral)
    isolated epidural lesions do occur, due to hematogenous spread, or from epidural lymphatics
    epidural disease—frequently results in clinically significant cord compression
- MR appearance
    epidural disease
        T_1—isointense to slightly hyperintense to cord
        T_2—hyperintense to cord
        homogeneous contrast enhancement
    vertebral disease
        T_1—inhomogeneous low SI
        T_2—intermediate or high SI

32.341

Leukemia

- most common malignancy of childhood; ninth most common malignancy in adults
- malignant proliferation of hematopoietic cells—arises in lymphoid tissue and bone marrow
- symptoms
    bone pain (pressure, rapidly proliferating cells)
- bone involvement most often diffuse, but can be focal (most common in acute myelogenous forms)
- CNS serves as sanctuary in chemotherapy, thus CNS frequent site of relapse

32.3452 (see also 33.3452)

Multiple myeloma

- neoplastic overgrowth of plasma cells
- one-third of bone malignancies
- peak incidence 50–70 years of age
- vertebral involvement most common in thoracic region
- sensitivity
    MR better than plain films and radionuclide bone scans
- MR appearance
    diffuse marrow infiltration most common
    nodular deposits within normal marrow can be seen

32.3631 (see also 31.3631)

Astrocytoma

- majority of intramedullary spinal cord tumors are either astrocytoma or ependymoma in type
- astrocytomas more common in children, ependymomas more common in adults
- imaging cannot differentiate astrocytoma from ependymoma
    involvement of entire width of cord, homogeneous high SI on T_2—favors astrocytoma
    small nodular tumor with cysts favors ependymoma
- three-fourths of astrocytomas—cervical or thoracic location

32.364 (see also 33.364)

Neurogenic tumors (nerve/nerve sheath origin tumors)

- incidence
    majority of thoracic spine paraspinal lesions (most common cause of posterior mediastinal mass)
    in adults, schwannomas and neurofibromas are most common (and have similar imaging characteristics)
    in young children, neuroblastoma is most common
- lesion type
    schwannomas = neurinomas = neurilemomas
        arise from Schwann cells of nerve root sheath
        extrinsic (eccentric) to nerve root
        imaging characteristics
            hypo- to isointense on T_1 to cord
            hyperintense on T_2, often heterogeneous (high SI areas = small cysts)
            heterogeneous enhancement, often more intense peripherally
    neurofibromas
        arise from Schwann cells, distinguished from schwannoma by abundant connective tissue and presence of nerve cells
        enlarge nerve itself
        usually associated with neurofibromatosis, even when solitary
        imaging characteristics
            homogeneous enhancement (may aid differentiation from schwannoma)
    tumors arising from primitive sympathetic neuroblasts (embryonic neural crest)—different types distinguished by degree of cellular maturation
        neuroblastoma
            malignant: undifferentiated neuroblasts
            majority arise from adrenals, remainder found along sympathetic chain

prognosis

>> worse with increasing age

>> better with spinal, than abdominal or pelvic lesions

> extradural extension common with paravertebral lesions

ganglioneuroblastoma

> malignant: undifferentiated neuroblasts and mature ganglion cells

ganglioneuroma

> benign: mature ganglion cells

> more common in adolescents and young adults

32.365

Arteriovenous malformation (AVM) and arteriovenous fistula (AVF)

- definition

> AVM—nidus of pathologic vessels between enlarged feeding arteries and draining veins

> AVF—arteries drain directly into enlarged veins

- types

> dural AVF (most common)

>> dorsal aspect of lower cord and conus

>> occur in elderly men

>> single transdural feeder

>> present with progressive neurologic deficits (venous stasis, infarction)

> intramedullary AVM

>> young patients

>> one cause of intramedullary hemorrhage

>> dorsal location, cervicomedullary region

>> multiple feeders lead to compact vascular plexus, which drains into tortuous venous plexus surrounding cord

>> present with acute hemorrhagic stroke

>> imaging appearance

>>> flow voids within cord

>>> enlarged extramedullary feeding vessels (typically anterior to cord)

> intradural extramedullary AVF

>> occur in third to sixth decades

>> anterior to cord, at conus level (most common), with supply by anterior spinal artery

>> present with progressive neurologic deficits

- imaging

> MR—important technique for initial diagnosis

>> large vessels identified as filling defects, best seen within cord on T_1 and in CSF on T_2

associated features—hemorrhage, edema, myelomalacia

small lesions best seen postcontrast (enhancement of venous component)

pitfall—CSF flow artifacts may mimic an AVM (on T_2)

myelography—filling defects due to enlarged vessels, cord atrophy

angiography—definitive diagnosis

intra-aortic injection, followed by selective vessel catheterization, assessing feeding vessels and venous drainage

Aneurysm

- usually associated with intramedullary AVM
- angiography—definitive study

32.3661 (see also 31.3661)

Meningioma

- incidence

    one third in cervical, two thirds in thoracic spine

    incidence rate of 1:3 (male: female)

    intradural location most common (but may be extradural)

- surgery

    complete removal achieved in 95%

    microsurgical technique important to minimize neurologic deficits

    with complete removal, 5% recur

- imaging appearance

    MR

    isointense with cord on T_1 and T_2

    marked contrast enhancement, with improved lesion identification

    capping inferiorly and superiorly by CSF—demonstrates lesion to be intradural, extramedullary (by far the most common location)

    plain film/CT

    dense calcification common

32.3662

Neuroenteric cyst

- embryology

    during early embryonic development, a temporary structure (canal of Kovalesvsky) connects amnion and primitive yolk sac

    persistence of canal leads to a fistula from gut, through vertebral bodies and cord, to dorsal skin

    persistence of portions of canal—origin of mesenteric cysts, enteric diverticula, neuroenteric cysts, diastematomyelia, spina bifida

- features (neuroenteric cysts)
    - enteric-lined cysts
    - located within spinal canal (can have component outside canal)
    - ventral to cord
    - location—cervicothoracic junction or conus medullaris
    - frequent associated vertebral body anomalies
- imaging appearance
    - MR
        - determined by blood and protein content, viscosity, pulsatility
    - differential diagnosis
        - arachnoid cyst—isointense to CSF on all sequences, no vertebral body anomalies

---

32.367

Subarachnoid hemorrhage

- most common cause—aneurysm or AVM of cord; may originate from cerebral source
- MR
    - acutely—moderate increase in CSF SI on T_1—obscures cord and nerve roots (not easily detected by MR)
    - subacutely—high T_1 SI (methemoglobin)

Epidural, subdural hemorrhage

- pathogenesis
    - lumbar puncture
    - trauma
    - hemorrhagic diathesis
    - anticoagulant therapy
    - vascular malformations
    - vasculitis
    - pregnancy
- imaging appearance
    - MR
        - SI—stage dependent
        - may be difficult to differentiate epidural vs. subdural location
    - differential diagnosis
        - angiolipoma
            - rare benign tumor
            - composed of lipocytes and abnormal blood vessels (latter causes hyperintensity on T_2—slow flow)
            - epidural location, midthoracic region
            - can cause bone erosion, pathologic fracture, cord compression
        - extradural lipomatosis (chronic steroid use, Cushing's disease)

32.369

Extramedullary hematopoiesis

- pathogenesis
    - compensatory response to insufficient red blood cell production by bone marrow
    - seen in thalassemia, hereditary spherocytosis, myelosclerosis
- anatomic involvement
    - favored sites—spleen, liver, lymph nodes
    - thoracic involvement
        - rare
        - usually asymptomatic
        - paraspinal mass—extrusion of proliferating marrow into subperiosteal location
        - intraspinal mass—represents extrusion of bone marrow, or development of marrow from embryonic hematopoietic rests
            - can cause cord compression
- imaging appearance
    - multiple, smoothly marginated, paraspinal masses
    - no bone erosion
    - SI of marrow
- differential diagnosis
    - lymphoma
    - metastatic disease

32.37 (see also 31.37, 33.37)

Leptomeningeal metastases

- pathogenesis
    - CNS tumors
        - glioblastoma
        - ependymoma
        - medulloblastoma
        - pineal tumors
    - nonCNS tumors
        - lung carcinoma
        - breast carcinoma
        - melanoma
        - lymphoma
- clinical presentation—varied
    - back pain
    - leg pain
    - headache
    - cranial, spinal nerve deficits
    - gait disturbance

- diagnosis

  CSF cytology—gold standard—may require multiple samples and large volume of CSF

  CT—nodular-filling defects within CSF, clumping of nerve roots

  MR—markedly improved sensitivity relative to CT when employed with IV-contrast enhancement

---

32.4113

Burst fracture

- axial loading injury
- vertical compression forces nucleus pulposus into vertebral body
- radial displacement of fragments
- most common: T9 to L5
- usually involve only one vertebral body, but frequently other injuries coexistent
- neurologic deficits occur due to retropulsed fragments
- CT—study of choice for initial evaluation
- MR—detects associated cord (edema, hemorrhage) and ligamentous injuries

---

32.458

Spinal cord ischemia/infarction

- etiology

  atherosclerosis

  vasculitis

  embolism

  infection

  surgery (abdominal aortic aneurysm resection)

  radiation

  trauma

- anatomical involvement

  central gray matter

  lower thoracic cord and conus (most common)

    supplied by artery of Adamkiewicz (usually arising from ninth to twelfth intercostal artery)

    blood flow is highest to this section of cord, given abundance of gray matter and its higher metabolic need

    region of cord most vulnerable to hypoperfusion

- MR—imaging modality of choice

  extent of abnormality—correlates well with clinical findings and prognosis

    anterior horn involvement only

    anterior and posterior horns involved, together with adjacent central white matter

    involvement of entire cord cross-section (severe disease)

T_2—high SI (vasogenic edema)

T_1—cord enlargement

contrast enhancement (disruption of blood-cord barrier secondary to ischemia)

can see associated marrow changes, also due to ischemia

differential diagnosis—vascular distribution (craniocaudal extent and in cross section) aids differentiation

> MS
>
> transverse myelitis
>
> neoplasia

32.783 (see also 31.783, 33.783)

Disk herniation—thoracic

- most common at lower four interspaces (where spine is more mobile)
- less common than cervical or lumbar herniation
- clinical presentation—often not clear cut

  back pain

  paresthesias

  motor weakness
- MR

  well demonstrates mass effect on cord, and contour deformity of cord

  must obtain whole spine localizer image (in addition to dedicated thoracic spine images), to correctly define level of disk herniation

  > MR markers—assist in correct level identification—vitamin E capsules, or oil (Johnson's baby oil) in a strip of IV tubing

  contrast enhancement—identifies dilated, engorged epidural venous plexus above and below herniated disk

---

32.861

Butterfly vertebra

- concave superior and inferior endplates, central osseous defect
- incidental finding of no clinical significance
- can be associated congenital abnormalities (diastematomyelia)

32.8613

Scoliosis

- lateral curvature of spine
- 90% idiopathic

  no underlying cause

  more common in females

  thoracic curvature is convex to right

  S-shaped curve

  progression beyond 50° necessitates surgery

- 10%—congenital, neuromuscular, post-traumatic
    - congenital
        - vertebral anomalies—butterfly vertebral body, hemivertebra
        - abnormalities of the cord
            - Chiari I, II malformation
            - syringohydromyelia
            - diastematomyelia
            - spinal cord neoplasm
    - neuromuscular—cerebral palsy—C-shaped curve
    - post-traumatic—fracture, old osteomyelitis, surgery, radiation therapy
- MR—imaging modality of choice for study of atypical or progressive scoliosis
    - utility of coronal plane (in conjunction with sagittal)
- plain films—quantitation of curvature (degree), and monitoring of progression

---

32.871

Multiple sclerosis (MS)

- see 31.871

32.89 (also 33.89)

Epidural lipomatosis

- excessive fat deposition in epidural space
- pathogenesis—chronic steroid use, morbid obesity
- 60% thoracic, 40% lumbar
- symptomatic patients—weakness, pain—due to compression of thecal sac

Lumbar Spine..

33.1214

Normal lumbar spine

- Anatomy
    - overview
        - five lumbar segments (vertebral bodies), five (fused) sacral segments, coccyx
        - intervertebral disks—central gelatinous core (nucleus pulposus, high SI on T_2 MR) with surrounding dense fibrous tissue (anulus fibrosus, low SI on T_1 and T_2 MR)
        - bony elements—pedicles, transverse processes, articular pillars (pars interarticularis, superior and inferior articular facets), laminae, spinous processes, vertebral body

facet joints—diarthrodial synovial-lined, richly innervated, on axial imaging superior articular facet forms "cap" anterolaterally with inferior articular facet posteromedial connecting to lamina

ligamentum flavum—extends from anterior aspect of upper lamina to posterior aspect of lower lamina

prominent epidural venous plexus

dermatomes—foot innervated by L4 (medial big toe), L5 (midfoot), and S1 (little toe)

sagittal plane

conus terminates (tip) between L1 and L2

posterior longitudinal ligament—posterior to vertebral bodies, anterior to thecal sac, 1 mm thick (anteroposterior), 5 mm wide (left to right)

facet joints of upper lumbar spine—oriented in sagittal plane, those of lower lumbar spine—more in coronal plane

parasagittal images—dorsal root ganglion (and ventral root) lies in superior portion of neural foramen

used for evaluation of foraminal stenosis

foramen—margins are disk and vertebral body anteriorly, pedicles superiorly and inferiorly, facet joints posteriorly

axial plane

bony canal—vertebral body anteriorly, pedicles laterally, lamina posteriorly

- T_1-weighted spin-echo imaging

normally hydrated (nondegenerated) disks—slightly hypointense to vertebral marrow

normal ligamentum flavum—well seen (intermediate SI)

4-mm sagittal (from pedicle to pedicle), 3-mm axial sections standard

anteriorly placed coronal saturation slab important to decrease artifacts from motion of anterior structures (used as well on T_2)

slices angled to be parallel to disk space

- T_2-weighted spin-echo imaging

normally hydrated (nondegenerated) disks—markedly hyperintense to vertebral marrow

in sagittal plane in adults, central band of low SI typically noted ("intranuclear cleft"), due to fibrous transformation

4-mm sagittal sections standard

fast T_2—replacing standard T_2 spin echo for routine clinical evaluation

- image normalization

surface coil imaging (standard for lumbar spine)—superficially located structures (close to coil) have artifactual high SI (= nonhomogeneous SI across FOV, unlike cylindrical coils used for head imaging)

typical window and center chosen for display of spinal canal leads to posterior structures being obscured (markedly hyperintense)

image normalization—postprocessing—attenuates signal from tissues close to coil, providing more homogeneous SI across FOV

33.12988

Contrast media

- normal-enhancing structures

    epidural venous plexus (nonfenestrated capillary endothelium, which confines contrast to intravascular space) = "Baston's plexus"

    basivertebral vein (central and posterior within vertebral body)

    dorsal root ganglion (fenestrated endothelium, present in muscle, marrow, and dorsal root ganglion—permits contrast to enter interstitial space)—enhancement is moderate in degree

- indications

    postoperative back

        differentiation of scar from disk

            on scans obtained within 20 min following contrast injection, scar enhances, recurrent (or residual) disk does not

    without previous surgery

        improved definition of disk-thecal sac interface

        identification of epidural venous plexus and (de novo) scar

        improved visualization of neural foramina

    neoplastic disease

        intradural

        soft tissue extradural involvement

    other disease processes involving the cord

        ischemia

        demyelination

    infection

33.13

Evolution of vertebral body and disk appearance

- infant

    absence of adult lumbar lordosis

    stage I (< 1 month of age)

        ossification center—low SI on T_1 and T_2

        slightly high T_1 SI band within ossification center—basivertebral venous plexus

        cartilaginous endplate—higher T_1 SI than paraspinous muscle, high T_2 SI

        disk—thin, isointense (T_1) to paraspinous muscle, highest T_2 SI

        anteroposterior dimension of ossification centers < intervertebral disks

    stage II (1–6 months of age)

        ossification center—low to intermediate SI on T_1, now isointense with endplates cartilaginous endplate—higher T_2 SI than muscle and ossification center

disk—low T_1, high T_2 SI

stage III (older than 7 months)—more adult appearance

ossification center— more rectangular, hyperintense on T_1 to muscle

cartilaginous endplate—T_1 and T_2 SI similar to ossification center

disk—low T_1 (isointense to muscle), high T_2 SI

conus

at birth, terminates above L3–4 level (termination below L3—abnormal regardless of age)

by 2 months of age, in adult location (L2–3 or above)

average position (child/adult)—L1–2

- young adult to elderly

vertebral body SI due to combination of red and yellow bone marrow—red (hematologically active) marrow has lower T_1 SI than yellow (fatty)

change in SI from infant to young adult and young adult to elderly reflects conversion from red to yellow bone marrow

with increasing age, both diffuse and focal replacement of red bone marrow by yellow bone marrow occurs

focal changes (focal "fat")—more common near endplates, perhaps due to decreased vascularity and earlier bone marrow conversion

---

33.131

Transitional vertebrae

- common anomaly of lumbosacral junction (4–8%)
- by definition, requires articulation or fusion of enlarged transverse process of lowest lumbar segment to sacrum
- on sagittal images, body of transitional segment may be square (normal configuration for lumbar), wedge-shaped (like sacral segments), or intermediate
- unilateral or bilateral
- known cause of back pain

decreased mobility at affected level

increased mobility and stress at interspace immediately above

---

33.133

Spina bifida occulta (occult spinal dysraphism)

- skin-covered developmental anomaly with incomplete midline closure, and no visible neural tissue or mass—includes diastematomyelia, dermal sinus tracts, fibrous bands, dermoids, neurenteric cysts, lipomas
- separate class (distinct) from meningoceles, myelomeningoceles
- not associated with Chiari II malformation

33.139

Schmorl's node

- prolapse of nucleus pulposus through endplate into medullary space of vertebral body (due to axial loading)
- typically asymptomatic
- imaging appearance
    - plain film—focal depression, contiguous with endplate, sclerotic rim
    - MR
        - T_1 lower, T_2 higher SI than marrow
        - often surrounding focal endplate changes
        - contrast enhancement (often peripheral) due to granulation tissue
        - utility of sagittal scans—demonstration of location immediately adjacent to disk space

33.141

Caudal regression (sacral agenesis)

- absence of sacrococcygeal vertebrae, with or without lumbar involvement
    - level of regression below L1 in most cases
    - agenesis limited to sacrum in half of all cases
- associated anomalies—cord tethering, renal dysplasia, pulmonary hypoplasia, neuromuscular weakness or paralysis
- associated with maternal diabetes
- imaging appearance
    - MR
        - wedge-shaped cord terminus in half (dorsal aspect extends further caudally than ventral aspect)
        - well depicts level of regression, presence of stenosis (in area of vertebral absence), vertebral anomalies

33.142 (see also 31.142)

Spinal stenosis

- congenital
    - short, thickened pedicles with a decreased interpediculate distance
    - decreased anteroposterior (<11.5 mm) and transverse dimensions of canal
    - tapering of canal in lumbar region (canal in anteroposterior dimension usually equal in size or greater to that in thoracic region)
    - may also have narrowed lateral recesses or neural foramina
    - predisposes patient to early degenerative disk disease
    - clinical presentation—typically myelopathic symptoms, but radicular symptoms may be present due to nerve root impingement

- degenerative
    - subtypes
        - central
        - lateral recess (subarticular canal)
            - definition—space between posterior margin of vertebral body and anterior margin of superior facet
            - anatomic bounds—thecal sac medially, pedicle laterally
            - size—> 5 mm, normal; < 3 mm, symptomatic
        - foraminal
    - cause
        - ligamentum flavum hypertrophy
            - anatomy
                - paired, thick, fibroelastic band (normal thickness = 3 mm in lumbar spine)
                - connects lamina of adjacent vertebral bodies
                - extends from anteroinferior aspect of superior lamina to posterosuperior aspect of inferior lamina
                - situated posterolaterally in canal
                - anterolaterally—contiguous with capsule of facet joint
            - pathology
                - with degenerative spine disease, becomes fibrotic, visibly thickened, buckled—narrows posterolateral canal (thus lateral recess), may also narrow central canal and/or neural foramina
        - facet joint hypertrophy
            - hypertrophy of superior articular facet is primary cause of lateral recess stenosis
            - failure to recognize lateral recess stenosis—major cause of persistent symptoms following lumbar diskectomy
        - neural foraminal stenosis
            - anatomy
                - bounded by pedicles superiorly and inferiorly, vertebral body and disk anteriorly, facets posteriorly
                - lumbar nerve root exits from lateral recess, enters neural foramen
            - pathology
                - most common at L4–5, L5–S1
                - degenerative disease of disk, endplates, posterior elements (facets) all contribute
                - most common cause—hypertrophy of superior facet
                - stenosis is accentuated if disk is narrowed
                - radicular symptoms (nerve root compression)
                - also pain from degenerated facet joints (which are richly innervated)
            - imaging
                - sagittal plane best
                - obliteration of normal fat surrounding nerve root

clinical presentation

>chronic pain—lower back, buttocks

>paresthesia or pain in posterolateral leg

>pain aggravated by standing, walking; relieved by rest (sitting, or lying down)—opposite of disk herniation, which is aggravated by sitting

>neurologic deficits minimal (vs. disk herniation, which also demonstrates positive straight leg test)

pathogenesis

>nerve root ischemia

33.1452

Myelomeningocele

- terminology

>spina bifida—incomplete closure of posterior bony elements, contents of spinal canal can extend through this defect (with tethering of cord)

>>meningocele—contains dura and arachnoid, neurologic defects uncommon with simple meningocele

>>myelomeningocele—contains neural tissue (within expanded posterior subarachnoid space)

>>>intrauterine ultrasound—open neural arch, flared posterior elements, Chiari II malformation (near 100% association)

>>>MR, CT usually obtained postoperatively, often with retethering of cord—wide dysraphic defect with CSF-filled sac covered by skin

- MR—modality of choice for evaluation of soft tissue elements in suspected spinal dysraphism

---

33.1453

Anterior sacral meningocele

- protrusion of dura and leptomeninges anteriorly through defect in sacrum
- imaging appearance

>plain film—semicircular erosion of sacrum ("scimitar sign")

>MR—isointense with CSF on all sequences

>myelography—pedicle connecting cyst and thecal sac can be obstructed by adhesions and cyst not filled with contrast

---

33.1454

Diastematomyelia

- splitting of spinal cord into two hemicords, each invested by pia

>each hemicord contains central canal and dorsal and ventral horns

>60%—hemicords are within one subarachnoid space and dural sac

40%—separate sacs, fibrous band or osteocartilaginous spur nearly always present at most inferior aspect of cleft

for detection of spur, gradient echo is better than T_2 spin echo which is better than T_1 spin echo (sensitivity)

85% with cleft between T9 and S1 (50% lumbar)

- associated anomalies

vertebral segmentation anomalies (common)—fusion (block vertebrae), hemivertebrae, butterfly vertebra

spina bifida (nearly always present)

orthopedic foot problems (half of patients)—clubfoot

hydromyelia

- clinical presentation

nonspecific symptoms, related to cord tethering

cutaneous stigmata in more than 50% (hairy patches, nevi, lipomas)

- imaging

importance of axial (and coronal) scans—on sagittal scans, the split cord can be overlooked

33.1455

Lipomyelomeningocele

- lipoma—firmly attached to dorsal surface of cord, which herniates through dysraphic spinal canal

20% of skin-covered lumbosacral masses

50% of occult spinal dysraphism

occur in lumbosacral region

differentiated from myelomeningocele by

1. presence of lipoma (attached to dorsal surface of neural placode)
2. intact overlying skin layer

lipoma merges with and is indistinguishable from subcutaneous fat

distal cord—tethered by lipoma

associated anomalies

butterfly vertebrae, other vertebral segmentation anomalies

sacral anomalies

maldevelopment of feet, scoliosis

- clinical presentation

before 6 months of age, fluctuant subcutaneous mass

progressive neurologic symptoms (if corrective surgery not performed)

lower extremity weakness

sensory loss

urinary incontinence

gait disturbance

occasionally undetected until adulthood (since lesion is skin-covered)

33.1463

Dorsal dermal sinus

- midline epithelial-lined tract—from skin inwards (variable distance), >50 % in lumbosacral region

    terminates in soft tissue, at dura, or within thecal sac

    cord tethering—common

    on skin—hairy nevus, hyperpigmented patch, or capillary angioma

    associated dermoid or epidermoid tumor at tract termination (half of patients)

- clinical presentation

    infection

    symptoms of compression (by tumor mass)

- diagnosis made by

    ultrasound

    CT—hyperdense sinus tract

    MR—when infected, IV-contrast enhancement improves delineation of sinus tract, particularly intraspinal portion

33.1481

Tethered cord

- congenital anomaly—conus medullaris held at abnormally low position

    cause

        short (tight) filum terminale

            age of presentation variable (adults present frequently with radiculopathy)

            normal filum ≤2 mm diameter

        intradural lumbosacral lipoma

        diastematomyelia

        delayed consequence of myelomeningocele repair

            in this instance, not all patients with evidence of tethering on imaging will be symptomatic

- clinical presentation (symptoms due to cord ischemia, caused by traction)—young child with progressive neurologic dysfunction

    gait difficulty

    motor and sensory loss in lower extremities

    bladder dysfunction

- imaging appearance

    cord extends without change in caliber to lumbosacral region, tethers posteriorly, associated lipoma, dysraphic posterior spinal elements

    hydromyelia may be present (ependymal-lined cavity)

        when small, usually not symptomatic

    MR

        T_1 images in all three orthogonal planes important for depiction of abnormal anatomy axial imaging superior to sagittal for determination of level of conus (on sagittal images, differentiation between conus medullaris and cauda equina can be difficult)

for diagnosis of retethering, presence of adhesions is best criteria

- surgical treatment

  early diagnosis and treatment—prevents urinary incontinence

  use of synthetic dural grafts—decreases incidence of retethering

  aim of surgery is to untether cord, arrest symptom progression

  following surgery, level of cord termination does not change

  lipomas—removed as completely as possible, with attention to release of tether

Terminal myelocystocele

- rare congenital cystic dilatation of caudal central spinal canal

  "trumpetlike" flaring of distal central canal (pial-lined CSF space, may be larger than accompanying meningocele)

  surrounding meningocele

  posterior bony defect

  associated anomalies of gastrointestinal and genitourinary tracts, and vertebral bodies common

---

33.1484

Spinal meningeal cysts

- diverticula of meningeal sac, nerve root sheath or arachnoid

  most likely congenital origin

  types

  - I—extradural, without nerve roots

    arachnoid cysts

    sacral meningoceles

  - II—extradural, with nerve roots

    Tarlov's perineural cysts = nerve root sleeve cysts = focal dilatation of nerve root sleeve

    nerves may be in cyst or in wall

    cyst communicates freely with thecal sac

    spinal nerve root diverticula

  - III—intradural

    arachnoid cysts (intradural)

- clinical presentation

  usually asymptomatic

- imaging appearance

  common in sacral area

  frequently large, multiple, bilateral

  can cause erosion, scalloping of vertebral body, pedicle, foramen

  MR—CSF SI on all pulse sequences

33.1485

Lumbosacral nerve root anomalies

- 1–3% of population
- usually L5, S1 roots unilaterally
- types

    I—conjoined root—most common—two roots arise from single root sleeve, but exit separately (in appropriate foramina)

    II—two roots exit through single foramen (may be one foramen without a root)

    III—anastomotic root connects two adjacent roots

- clinical relevance

    asymptomatic

    potential for failed back surgery when accompanying disk herniation—requires adequate decompression

    can be mistaken on CT (without intrathecal contrast) for herniated disk

33.149

Fatty filum terminale

- normal filum terminale

    runs from tip of conus medullaris to end of thecal sac, inserts on first coccygeal segment

    ≤ 2 mm diameter at L5–S1 level

- 1–5% of patients—small amount of fat within filum terminale

    may be incidental or associated with cord tethering

33.1521

Achondroplasia

- pathogenesis

    autosomal dominant

    disorder of enchondral bone formation

    premature synostosis of ossification centers of vertebral bodies

- imaging appearance

    cervical spine

    in childhood, cervical changes may dominate presentation—canal narrowing, foramen magnum constriction

    lumbar spine

    thick, short pedicles

    interpedicular distance decreases from L1 to L5

    stenotic canal, predisposed to disk herniation

    accentuated lumbar lordosis, horizontal sacrum

33.1831

Neurofibromatosis

- see 31.1831

33.25

Disk space infection

- clinical presentation (postoperative)
    - severe back pain—1 to 4 weeks after surgery
    - fever, wound infection, elevation of white blood cells—seen in minority of patients
    - delays in diagnosis common
- pathogenesis
    - hematogenous seeding
        - children—disk is richly vascularized, serves as initial site of infection
        - adults—initial site of infection is vertebrae (subchondral portion) or soft tissue
    - postoperative (1–3% of back surgery patients)
        - *Staphylococcus aureus*—most common organism
- plain film
    - disk space narrowing, poorly defined endplates, sclerosis of adjacent vertebrae (all late changes)
- CT
    - disk space narrowing, cortical bone loss (endplate), paraspinous soft tissue mass (all late changes)
- MR
    - narrowed irregular disk, with high SI on T_2
    - high T_2 SI (low T_1 SI) of adjacent vertebral endplates—due to edema, inflammation—forms a horizontal band involving one third to one half of vertebral body
        - must be differentiated from degenerative type I endplate changes
    - contrast enhancement of endplates, disk space
    - indistinct vertebral endplates
    - paraspinous soft tissue mass—which enhances postcontrast
- radionuclide bone scan—sensitive, nonspecific

33.27

Arachnoiditis

- clumping, thickening of nerve roots
- initially a minimal cellular inflammatory response, which progresses to collagenous adhesions
- pathogenesis

infection (uncommon today)

previous surgery

hemorrhage

pantopaque

- CT (with moderate involvement)

nodular or cordlike intradural masses

nerve roots can be adherent to dura

- MR

three patterns

conglomerations of nerve roots centrally within thecal sac (mild disease)

adherence of nerve roots to periphery of thecal sac

increased soft tissue filling majority of thecal sac, no discernible individual nerve roots (severe disease)

pitfall—spinal stenosis can lead to false impression of nerve root clumping

when acute (meningitis)—contrast enhancement

- myelography

mild involvement—blunting of nerve root sleeves, fusion of nerve roots, irregularities along margin of thecal sac

moderate involvement—obliteration of nerve root sleeves, multisegmental fusion of nerve roots, adhesions, scarring of thecal sac, loculation

---

33.3122

Osteoid osteoma

- common benign skeletal neoplasm
- central nidus of osteoid, woven bone, fibrovascular tissue; < 2.0 cm diameter
- sharply demarcated from surrounding bone, variable surrounding osteosclerosis
- usually occurs in young patient, with pain relieved by aspirin; scoliosis common
- 10% in spine, here most common in neural arch of lumbar vertebra
- bone scintigraphy—focal activity (immediate and delayed images)
- CT—sclerosis surrounding lytic lesion, may demonstrate central calcified nidus

---

33.3123

Osteoblastoma = giant (> 2 cm) osteoid osteoma

- 40% of osteoblastomas located in spine (cervical, thoracic, lumbar)
- pain—presenting symptom
- often enlarge

33.3141

Vertebral body hemangioma

- benign neoplasm, common incidental finding on MR
- on autopsy series, found in 11% of patients
- solitary (most common) or multiple
- variable size—from small to involve entire vertebral body—posterior extension can cause canal compromise
- weakening of vertebral body can result in fracture
- histologic appearance—mixture of adipose and angiomatous tissue between prominent trabeculae
- plain film

    lytic foci with trabeculation

    thick vertical striation/trabeculation
- CT

    lucent lesion with "polka dot" densities that represent coarse vertical trabeculation
- MR

    focal region of high SI on T_1 and T_2

    reticular pattern of low SI—thickened trabeculae (prominent vertically)

    differential diagnosis—focal fat (within vertebral bodies)—which follows SI of fat on all sequences
- angiography—intense hypervascular stain

33.3182

Giant cell tumor

- rare (vertebral), with most common location being sacrum
- present between 20 and 40 years of age, female predominance
- better prognosis than giant cell tumors elsewhere in body, with low recurrence rate following resection
- lytic, expansile, aggressive, rarely crosses periosteum
- quite vascular, demonstrate contrast enhancement
- differential diagnosis—osteoblastoma (more common in posterior elements, less lobular), aneurysmal bone cyst (younger age group), metastatic disease
- MR

    lobular, intermediate T_1 SI, mixed T_2 SI

    high SI foci on T_2—hemorrhage, cystic regions

    low SI rim on both T_1 and T_2—sclerotic bone at tumor margin

33.319

Focal fat deposits (in vertebral marrow)

- pathogenesis—focal marrow ischemia, with fatty replacement of hematopoietic marrow

- can occur at any level in spine, frequently seen in multiple vertebral bodies
- round, up to 15 mm diameter
- more common in elderly patients (seen in > 90% of patients over 50 years of age on MR)
- MR—follow fat SI on all imaging sequences

33.327

Chordoma

- locally invasive, destructive, lytic, lobular, slow-growing
    calcification in half of all cases
    mixed solid and cystic components common
- location—50% sacrum/coccyx, 35% skull base (clivus), 15% vertebral body

---

33.33 (see also 31.33, 32.33)

Lumbar metastases

- vertebral column—most common site of skeletal metastatic disease
- etiology—lung cancer (most common), others—breast, prostate, renal cell, hematologic malignancies
- most cases of epidural compression of cord or cauda equina—due to vertebral metastasis with either bony collapse or posterior extension
    most patients—compression at only one level
- clinical presentation
    back pain (majority of patients)
    motor impairment (usually precedes sensory deficits)
    radiculopathy (uncommon)—compression of single nerve root can occur, mimicking disk herniation
- plain film
    absent pedicle—classic finding
- myelography
    high risk in patients with block (neurologic deterioration in up to one fourth)
    lesions above level of block easily missed
- MR (more sensitive than bone scintigraphy for vertebral metastases)
    vertebral body nearly always initial site of involvement
    sagittal imaging—provides screening of area of interest
    modality of choice for evaluation of epidural involvement (importance of axial imaging)
    contrast enhancement—useful for improved demonstration of epidural and soft tissue extent
    osteoblastic metastases (common with prostate carcinoma)—low SI on T_1 and T_2 (sclerosis on plain film)
        lung, breast carcinoma—typically lytic, but may be osteoblastic when treated

33.3452 (see also 32.3452)

Plasma cell myeloma

- malignant disease of plasma cells—includes both multiple myeloma and plasmacytoma
- plasmacytoma—single lesion of bone
    laboratory studies (blood)—may be positive or negative
    additional lesions may develop with time
    spine, pelvis—most common location
    osteolytic, expansile

33.362

Dermoid, epidermoid

- "pearly tumors" (gross appearance)
- presence of hair/skin elements—defines dermoid
- in spine, most involve lumbosacral region (with dermoids more common)
    intra- or extramedullary
    well-defined, rounded lesions—cystic portion contains desquamated epithelium and sebaceous gland secretions
    dermal sinus, spinal dysraphism—frequently associated

Teratoma

- rare in spinal canal, except for sacrococcygeal form (which can undergo malignant transformation, and is the most common presacral mass in a child)
- composed of tissue from all three germinal layers

Lymphangioma

- congenital lesion—obstruction of lymphatic drainage
- 75% in the neck (posterior triangle)—in this location, more common in children under 2 years
- typically asymptomatic, treated by surgical resection
- MR—low SI on T_1, high SI on T_2 (fluid)—septae and/or fat may be present between fluid spaces

33.3636

Ependymoma

- slow-growing, well-circumscribed, benign (complete surgical resection possible)
- 60–70% of all spinal cord tumors
- third to sixth decades of life
- majority arise in conus, cauda equina, or filum terminale (cervical cord—most common site for intramedullary ependymoma)

clinical presentation—nonspecific—motor, sensory deficits, sphincter dysfunction

- MR

    focal cord enlargement limited to two or three levels favors ependymoma over astrocytoma

    virtually all enhance strongly following contrast injection

---

33.364 (see also 32.364)

Neurofibroma, schwannoma

- most common of the nerve root sheath tumors
- majority intradural, extramedullary in location (one third—extradural)
- foraminal lesion may be mistaken for herniated disk—enhancement postcontrast allows differentiation
- differentiation

    schwannoma

        typically solitary

        well-circumscribed, eccentric to nerve

        heterogeneous on T_2

    neurofibroma

        multiplicity favors diagnosis

        fusiform enlargement of nerve

        homogeneous SI on T_2, may have target appearance (high SI peripherally, lower SI centrally)

33.369

Intradural lipoma

- on benign end of spectrum that includes lipomyelomeningocele
- dorsal spinal defect—minimal, if present
- developmental origin—premature separation of cutaneous ectoderm from neuroectoderm, with mesenchyme entering neural tube (later differentiating into fat)
- 1% of intraspinal tumors
- most lie along dorsal aspect of cord
- MR

    fat SI on all sequences

    chemical shift artifact along frequency-encoding direction (at interface of fat and CSF)

    nerve roots can in some cases be identified coursing through lesion

---

33.37 (see also 31.37, 32.37)

Leptomeningeal metastases

- poor patient prognosis

- one third of patients with metastases to brain or spine will develop leptomeningeal metastatic disease
- breast and lung carcinoma—most common visceral neoplasms to spread to subarachnoid space
- imaging appearance (lumbar)

  large and small nodules

  coating of nerve roots (and cord)—can be "beaded" in appearance

  intramedullary extension (rare)
- differential diagnosis

  infectious meningitis (immunosuppressed patients)

  toxoplasmosis

  sarcoidosis (cord involvement usually dominates)
- contrast-enhanced MR superior to CT myelography for detection

33.411

Flexion injury (lumbar spine)

- with lap belt (seat belt without shoulder strap), principal bony injury is lumbar spine fracture (Chance fracture)—flexion occurs (fulcrum) centered on anterior abdominal wall

  most commonly involves L2 or L3

  horizontal fracture (posterior elements)—but this need not be present

  distraction injury (ligamentous disruption) with little or no anterior vertebral body compression—may be unstable
- unrestrained occupant—flexion occurs (fulcrum) centered on posterior vertebral body

  anterior body compression fracture

  distraction of posterior elements

  most common at thoracolumbar junction

33.416

Pathologic compression fracture

- MR

  low T_1 SI, high T_2 SI—with complete replacement of normal marrow SI, may extend into pedicle

  most patients have multiple lesions in other vertebral bodies—round to oval in appearance (value of sagittal T_1 images for screening)

  offers valuable information regarding epidural extension, canal compromise

33.417

Osteoporotic compression fracture

- in elderly, due to insufficiency of bone (senile osteoporosis)
- more common in postmenopausal women

- MR

    acute—areas of low T_1 SI, high T_2 SI, but with areas of preserved, normal marrow

    chronic—signal isointense to normal marrow

33.423

Spondylolysis, spondylolisthesis

- spondylolysis—interruption of pars interarticularis

    unilateral or bilateral

        bilateral—allows motion of posterior elements relative to adjacent vertebrae—superior and inferior facets at involved level move independently

            superior facet remains attached to vertebral body

            inferior facet articulates and moves with more inferior level

    CT—defects seen on axial images as lucent clefts, oriented in coronal plane

    MR—discontinuity of bone difficult to visualize on axial images (best seen on parasagittal images)

    single photon emission tomography (SPECT) bone scintigraphy may identify traumatic lesions not seen on plain film or planar imaging

- spondylolisthesis—forward slippage of one vertebral body relative to adjacent more inferior body

    causes—post-traumatic/surgical, degenerative (facet joints), congenital

    narrows neural foramen (foramen assumes more horizontal orientation on sagittal images), may cause nerve root impingement

    canal narrowing—seen with degenerative type

    grading (degree of subluxation)

        I—up to one fourth of vertebral body

        II—one fourth to one half

        III—one half to three fourths

        IV—> three fourths

33.4239

Retrolisthesis

- posterior subluxation of vertebral body relative to adjacent inferior body
- caused by disk degeneration with preservation of facet joints
- following surgery or other intervention, with resultant neural foraminal narrowing (and nerve root impingement) is one cause of failed back syndrome
- most common in lumbar and cervical spine

    lumbar spine

        L3–4, L4–5 most commonly involved

        frequently accompanied by disk bulges, spurs

central canal stenosis—uncommon

neural foraminal narrowing—common

33.452

Pseudomeningocele

- tear in dura, with (most common) or without tear in arachnoid membrane
- variable size connection to subarachnoid space
- postlaminectomy—lesions most common in cervical spine (especially following surgery involving occiput), rare in lumbar spine (where they can produce radicular symptoms)

33.453

Postoperative—disk surgery

- postoperative scar

  homogeneous enhancement (due to intrinsic vascularity) on MR following IV-contrast administration (not consistently seen until > 3 months following surgery)

  one cause of persistent pain following lumbar disk surgery (re-operation contraindicated)

- recurrent or residual disk herniation

  no enhancement on MR obtained within 20 min following IV-contrast administration (mandates use of thin sections—≤ 3 mm to avoid partial volume effects)

  focal, smooth posterior protrusion of soft tissue, contiguous with native disk

  presence of mass effect favors diagnosis (vs. scar)

- other findings (MR postcontrast)

  decompressed nerve may enhance (should resolve by 6 months)

  facet joints may enhance—presumably due to surgical manipulation (can persist long term)

Failed back surgery syndrome

- recurrent symptoms following surgery (10–40% of patients)
- causative factors—recurrent disk herniation, spinal stenosis, arachnoiditis, epidural fibrosis

---

33.74

Ankylosing spondylitis

- inflammatory disease of unknown etiology
- sacroiliac joints involved early in disease course

  erosion of cortical margins with subchondral bony sclerosis first seen

  widening of joint space follows (bony erosion)

  fusion (obliteration) of sacroiliac joints—end result

- spine

    inflammation—at junction of anulus fibrosis and vertebral body

    outer annular fibers become replaced by bone—syndesmophytes which eventually bridge adjacent vertebral bodies

    advanced disease—"bamboo spine"

    complications—fracture with minor trauma, in cervical spine can lead to quadriplegia

---

33.779

Synovial cyst

- associated with facet degenerative changes
- clinical presentation—radicular pain, often sciatic (can mimic disk herniation)

    can compress thecal sac

- imaging appearance

    CT—cystic (hypo- to hyperdense), may be calcified, adjacent to facet joint

    MR—SI appearance of fluid variable, enhancement of solid component and cyst capsule (delayed enhancement of cyst)

    recognition of relationship to facet joint important for diagnosis

---

33.781

Degenerative disk and endplate changes

- disk

    MR

    > loss of disk height

    > annular tears

    > decreased T_2 SI (most sensitive indicator of early disk degeneration)—due to decrease in proteoglycans and in ratio of chondroitin sulfate B to keratin sulfate

    > with exception of trauma, disk herniation without changes of disk degeneration is very unusual

- endplate

    changes are parallel and directly adjacent to disk space

    changes typically involve the entirety of both endplates, although involvement of just one endplate (and even just a portion of one) can occur

    MR

    > type I

    >> increased water content, with decreased SI on T_1, and increased SI on T_2

    >> enhance on T_1 (often to isointensity with marrow fat) postcontrast

    >> differential diagnosis

metastatic disease—typically there are multiple lesions, with isolated involvement of endplate uncommon

disk space infection/osteomyelitis—involvement of disk in addition to adjacent vertebral bodies, demarcation between disk and body lost, presence of paraspinous mass

type II

fatty infiltration—increased T_1 and T_2 SI paralleling fat

temporal progression of type I to II has been observed

mixed type I and II patterns occur

type III (rare)

bony sclerosis—low SI on both T_1 and T_2

Spondylosis = degenerative disease of the spine

- common findings include osteophytes, Schmorl's nodes, endplate sclerosis

to be differentiated from:
Syndesmophytes

- slender, vertical ligamentous calcification extending from osseous excrescence of one vertebral body to next
- hallmark of ankylosing spondylitis

33.782

Vacuum intervertebral disk

- degenerated disk with gas (nitrogen) in clefts of anulus fibrosis and nucleus pulposus
- more common in lumbar spine and in elderly patients
- CT—very low density collections within disk
- MR—linear low SI on T_1 and T_2 (gas = signal void)

33.783 (see also 31.783, 32.783)

Disk bulge, protrusion, extrusion (disk herniation)

- tears of anulus fibrosus

classification

concentric (type I)—parallel to curvature of outer disk

radial (type II)—involve all layers of anulus from nucleus to surface

transverse (type III)—involve insertion of Sharpey's fibers into ring apophysis

high SI on T_2

enhancement following IV gadolinium chelate administration (due to presence of fibrovascular tissue = granulation tissue from normal reparative process)

- disk (annular) bulge

    posterior disk margin—smooth curvilinear contour—extending beyond margin of adjacent vertebral endplates—without focal disk protrusion

    broad-based, circumferential

    occurs early in disk degeneration

    due to laxity of and tears within anulus fibrosus

    can narrow spinal canal and inferior neural foramen

- disk protrusion

    herniation of nucleus through (small) tear in anulus, contained by outer fibers of anulus

    differentiated from bulge by axial imaging—focal extension of disk material beyond margin of vertebral endplates

    most common posteriorly and laterally

- disk extrusion

    herniation of nucleus through ruptured anulus

    extruded material remains in contiguity with parent disk

    even without surgery, granulation tissue (which enhances postcontrast on MR) forms surrounding disk

    substantial reduction in size of disk herniation can be observed with conservative therapy

    when combined with lateral stenosis, can cause nerve root ischemia with eventual fibrosis, leading to irreversible axonal damage location

    90% of lumbar lesions occur at L4–5 or L5–S1, majority of remainder at L3–4

    central—may cause no symptoms—exiting nerve roots unaffected

    paracentral—causes symptoms due to compression of exiting nerve root (for example, S1 with an L5–S1 disk extrusion)

    lateral

    least common (anulus is thinnest posteriorly)

    more often present at L2–3, L3–4

    superior migration of fragments common

    compress ganglion or nerve root within neural foramen (radiculopathy of nerve root above interspace—for example L3 with an L3–4 disk extrusion)

    occur beyond termination of nerve root sleeve, thus myelography is relatively insensitive exam

    myelographic findings—displacement of contrast-filled sac; elevation, displacement, or amputation of nerve root sleeve; nerve root enlargement (edema)

- free fragment (sequestered disk)

    herniated disk material is separate from parent disk

    may be anterior (contained by) or posterior to posterior longitudinal ligament (when anterior, a thin midline septum directs fragments into paracentral region away from midline) can migrate superiorly or inferiorly within epidural space, or into neural foramen

MR

    low to intermediate T_1 SI

    high T_2 SI ($\leq$CSF)

- lumbar nerve root enhancement (MR)

    origin—disruption of blood-nerve root barrier

    presence—supports clinical significance of a compressing lesion

---

33.84

Paget's disease

- bone destruction (lysis) followed by attempts at repair

    lytic phase—bone resorption, with replacement of marrow by vascular fibrous connective tissue

    reparative phase—resorbed bone replaced by dense irregular new bone

- clinical presentation

    commonly asymptomatic

    dull pain

    spinal stenosis with neurologic dysfunction

- osteogenic sarcoma—< 1%
- imaging appearance (general)—cortical thickening, coarse trabeculae, bone expansion, areas of lucency, evidence of bone softening
- plain film—findings noted in skull, spine, pelvis, long bones

    skull—osteoporosis circumscripta—sharply demarcated area of radiolucency in which bone is ill-defined

    spine

        thickened cortex

        thickened, irregular, coarse vertical-oriented trabeculae

    long bones

        bowing

        insufficiency (stress) fractures—transverse

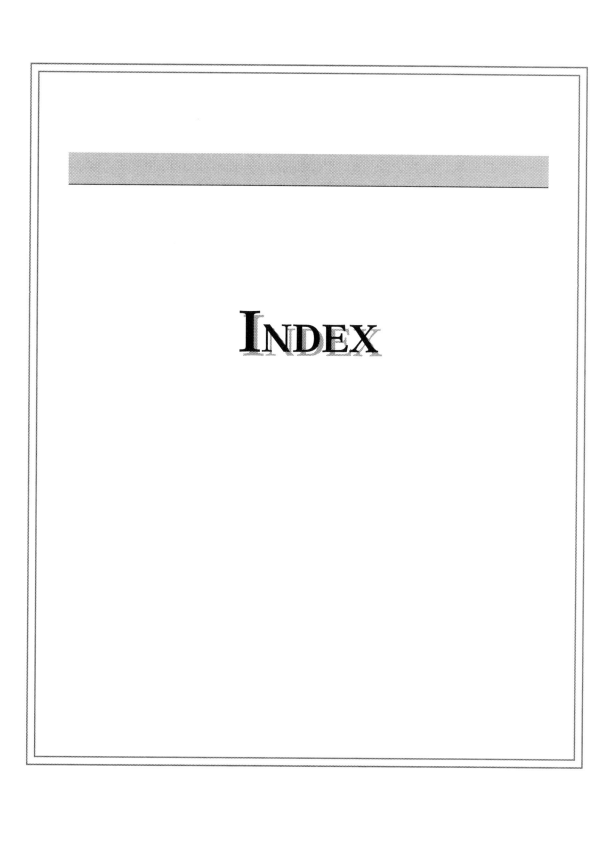

INDEX